The Economics of Social Capital and Health

A Conceptual and Empirical Roadmap

World Scientific Series in Global Healthcare Economics and Public Policy

ISSN: 2010-2089

Series Editor-in-Chief: Richard M Scheffler
University of California, Berkeley, USA

Published:

World Scientific Series in Global Healthcare Economics and Public Policy – Vol. 2

The Economics of Social Capital and Health

A Conceptual and Empirical Roadmap

Edited by

Sherman Folland
Oakland University, USA

Lorenzo Rocco
University of Padova, Italy

Foreword by

Richard M. Scheffler
University of California, Berkeley

W World Scientific

NEW JERSEY · LONDON · SINGAPORE · BEIJING · SHANGHAI · HONG KONG · TAIPEI · CHENNAI

Published by

World Scientific Publishing Co. Pte. Ltd.
5 Toh Tuck Link, Singapore 596224
USA office: 27 Warren Street, Suite 401-402, Hackensack, NJ 07601
UK office: 57 Shelton Street, Covent Garden, London WC2H 9HE

Library of Congress Cataloging-in-Publication Data
Folland, Sherman, author.
    The economics of social capital and health : a conceptual and empirical roadmap /
Sherman Folland and Lorenzo Rocco.
        p. ; cm. -- (World Scientific series in global healthcare economics and public policy ;
volume 2)
    Includes bibliographical references and index.
    ISBN 978-9814293396 (hardcover : alk. paper)
    I. Rocco, Lorenzo, 1975- author. II. Title. III. Series: World Scientific series in global healthcare
economics and public policy ; v. 2. 2010-2089
    [DNLM: 1. Public Health--economics. 2. Community Networks--economics. 3. Health
Promotion--economics. 4. Social Networking. WA 30]
    RA410.5
    362.1--dc23
                                                                    2013041078

British Library Cataloguing-in-Publication Data
A catalogue record for this book is available from the British Library.

In-house Editor: Chye Shu Wen

Typeset by Stallion Press
Email: enquiries@stallionpress.com

Printed in Singapore by World Scientific Printers.

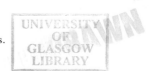

This volume has been an excellent opportunity for the building of social capital, and is dedicated to the many people who contributed in many ways to its creation.

Foreword

This book contains cutting-edge theoretical and empirical thinking on the relationship between social capital and health. The distinctive feature of this book is that its contributions are made by economists whose points of view differ from those of others who have contributed to this literature. The book seeks to address six questions, the answers to which are unique contributions to understanding the relationship between social capital and health:

1. What do economists working in the health arena bring to the intellectual debate on social capital that others have not?
2. What do economists have to offer to the understanding of the possible links and relationships between social capital and health?
3. Which paradigms in economics are the most useful in understanding the possible links and relationships between social capital and health?
4. What have economists studied empirically? What are the weaknesses of these studies?
5. How do economists attempt to overcome the weaknesses in their empirical work?
6. What factors contribute to the social capital and health relationship?

This book begins by laying out the theoretical foundations between social capital and health. Chapters 1–5 focus on the theoretical and conceptual issues, while Chapters 6–10 focus on the empirical and policy relationships between social capital and health. Readers will think differently and more deeply about the relationship between social capital and health after reading this book.

Richard M. Scheffler
Distinguished Professor of Health Economics
University of California, Berkeley
January 2014

About the Contributors

Sherman Folland attained a Ph.D in Health Economics at the University of Iowa in 1975. He is presently Professor at Oakland University in Michigan. He and his wife, Donna, have two cherished daughters now in their twenties. Folland has published over 30 articles in *Health Economics*; *Journal of Health Economics*; *Health Economics, Policy and Law*; *Social Science & Medicine* and others. His earlier work covering a variety of topics proved useful for his contributions to the successful, co-authored textbook *The Economics of Health and Health Care*. For the past 10 years, he has researched solely on questions in the economics of social capital and health, especially working on causality issues and efforts to improve the theory.

Lorenzo Rocco attained a Ph.D in economics at the University of Toulouse I, France, in 2005 before moving back to Italy where he is currently Assistant Professor of Economics at the University of Padova. He is an empirical economist and his fields of research include the socio-economic determinants of health, the influence of health on the labor market outcomes and several aspects of the economics of education. His research has been published in *The Economic Journal*, *Health Economics*, *Public Choice* among others. He has also contributed to several reports commissioned by the World Bank, World Health Organization and The European Commission.

Eline Aas is Associate Professor in Health Economics at the Department of Health Management and Health Economics at the University of Oslo, and has an honorary contract with the University of York. Aas' research is related to inequalities in health, social capital on health, estimation of health care costs and economic evaluation.

José Anchorena attained a Ph.D in Economics, Carnegie Mellon University. His main interests are economic development, macroeconomics, public policy and economic history. He has been visiting researcher at University of Oslo and is presently Director of Economic Development at Fundación Pensar, Argentina.

Yumna Bahgat attained a B.A. in Social Welfare with a minor in Global Poverty and Practice at the University of California, Berkeley. She is a researcher at the Nicholas C. Petris Center of Health Care Markets and Consumer Research and has worked on the Berkeley Forum Report project.

Beatrice d'Hombres works at the Joint Research Center of the European Commission (Unit of Econometrics and Applied Statistics). She has been with the Joint Research Center since 2006 and she holds a Ph.D in Economics from the University of Clermont-Ferrand, France. Her research interests are in education and health economics as well as in applied econometrics.

Elena Fumagalli holds a Ph.D in Economics from the University of Venice and she is now a post-doctorate at the University of Lausanne. She has worked at the University of East Anglia and she has been consultant for the European Commission. She is interested in economics of aging, risky behaviors, social capital/social networks and the evaluation of public policies.

Kamrul Islam is a senior researcher at Uni Rokkan Centre in Bergen, Norway. He obtained his Ph.D in Health Economics from Lund University, Sweden in 2007, and MSc in Health Economics from the University of York, in 2000. Dr. Islam has extensive experience with cross-disciplinary research and he has published his research in reputed international journals.

Tor Iversen is Professor of Health Economics at the University of Oslo, Norway. His research interests include social capital and health, the role of economic incentives in health care and comparative health system research.

Oddvar Kaarbøe is Professor of Economics at the University of Bergen. He is also the research director of Health Economics Bergen (HEB). His main research area is the financing of health care institutions.

Audrey Laporte is an Associate Professor of Health Economics at the Institute for Health Policy, Management and Evaluation at the University of Toronto. Her work in the area of social capital has looked at the various ways that it can influence both health outcomes at a population level and health, and health care utilization at the individual level.

Sachiko Ozawa is an Assistant Scientist at Johns Hopkins Bloomberg School of Public Health in the Department of International Health. She applies health economic methods to improve health systems in low- and middle-income countries.

Her current research focuses on vaccines, health insurance, and the role of trust/social capital in health care.

Lucas Ronconi is a development economist working at the Centro de Investigación y Acción Social (CIAS) in Argentina. He received a Ph.D from the University of California Berkeley, a Fulbright scholarship, and a medal from the Global Development Network (GDN). His research has been published in several journals including *Economics Letters*, *Health Economics*, and *Industrial Relations*.

Richard M. Scheffler is Distinguished Professor of Health Economics and Public Policy at the School of Public Health and the Goldman School of Public Policy at the University of California, Berkeley. He also holds the Chair in Health Care Markets & Consumer Welfare endowed by the Office of the Attorney General for the State of California. Professor Scheffler is Director of The Nicholas C. Petris Center on Health Care Markets and Consumer Welfare. Professor Scheffler has published over 150 papers and edited and written six books. He has conducted a recent review on Pay For Performance in Health for the World Health Organization and the OECD. He is also Vice Chair of the Berkeley Forum for Improving California's Healthcare Delivery System and the lead author of the Berkeley Forum Report.

Contents

Chapter 1

Introduction to the Economics of Social Capital and Health

Sherman Folland and Lorenzo Rocco

Research on social capital strongly suggests that social interaction benefits society substantially. Its association with good health has attracted health economists to explore how this relationship arises and to develop econometric tests of social capital effects. The present book explores how and what health economists can contribute to this multidisciplinary undertaking. Our efforts are meant to complement what has gone before in the fields of economics, sociology, epidemiology, and others.

As papers from economist Glenn Loury (1977), sociologist James Coleman (1988), sociologist Pierre Bourdieu (1985), political scientist Robert Putnam (2000, 1995), and epidemiologist Ichiro Kawachi (1999) demonstrate, social capital came into being as an interdisciplinary branch of study. Among these writers, Putnam and Kawachi sought and found beneficial associations of social capital with health, and health economists now energetically pursue research on this relationship. The purpose of this book is to add value to this inheritance, to build on it, and to extend it using the tools of economics. We welcome the contributions of economists and researchers from other disciplines, and we hope that we offer a quick start for those unfamiliar with the subject. The chapters develop independently and can be read in any order.

Can economic analysis contribute to social capital research? Our answer is clearly positive, because economics emphasizes training and experience in model building and econometrics, areas that need development in social capital and health research. The potential gains are twofold: (1) A better understanding of how the elements of social capital interact with the rest of the economy; and (2) better coefficient estimates for the effects of social capital. The present volume is organized into two areas: theory and empirics.

The economists who have become intrigued with social capital include many of our most noted scholars. Gary Becker and Kevin Murphy (2000) developed a theory of decision making that is influenced by the purchasing choices of social majorities. George Akerlof (1998) studied the effects of marriage bonds on unhealthful behaviors. Edward Glaeser, David Laibson, and Bruce Sacerdote (2002) developed a dynamic model of social capital that predicts the lifecycle of memberships in social clubs. The social impact of income inequality is the theme of Joseph Stiglitz's 2012 book, "The Price of Inequality: How Today's Divided Society Endangers Our Future." Econometric criticisms and analysis of existing work by Steven Durlauf (2002) inspired health economic studies to develop means by which to identify the effects of social capital. Finally, the central role of trust in social capital research owes much to the insights of Kenneth Arrow (1975).

What are the Potential Benefits?

Economists may appreciate the opportunity to use their economic skills to benefit the course of interdisciplinary analysis, perhaps to clarify the complexity of the models, and to improve the sophistication of the statistical analysis. The social capital hypothesis suggests that social capital's benefits for the community may be substantial, perhaps radically so, but strong claims require strong evidence. As with other scientists, part of our commitment is to "blow the whistle" on the hypothesis should the results prove consistently negative, but a solid case appears to be developing in support of the public energy and resources necessary to improve a community's social capital.

What are the benefits to the community? Some communities, states, countries, and regions practice higher levels of social interaction than others, and we often also find in these areas higher levels of the "good" social outcomes, such as health, whether measured by self-reports, diagnostics, or mortality rates. These associations are also found at the individual level. Recently econometrics to determine the direction of the social capital effects has tended to find the relationship to be bidirectional: Increased increments of social capital improve health, and health increments tend to improve social participation. A simple question — do you find that other people can be trusted? — is closely associated with health and other beneficial social outcomes.

What is the best possible result? Inner-city and similar poverty areas, many of which have elevated crime, poor treatment of children, poor education outcomes, and poor health indicators, are unlikely lack only per capita income; income inequality and weak social capital may work as contributing and (possibly) controllable factors. The social capital and health hypothesis connects intrinsically to the thinking of every social observer who has sought to enhance the speed of community improvement.

This Book and Its Contributions

We first introduce the inherited theory. While economists often prefer to define social capital as a social network, a review of its intellectual history explains how the phrase came to have a more heterogeneous composition.

The literature typically depicts four pathways by which social capital affects health: Providing and sharing information, providing emotional support, instilling a sense of responsibility to others and to oneself, and generating organizations to promote community health resources.

During the current early stages of theory development related to social capital, researchers gather the elements that are associated with or interfere with its production. For example, social capital may interact with consumer goods that are good or bad for health. If social capital has an opportunity cost, then its effects will be felt through budget constraints. Social participation affects everything else in complex ways, and we must understand these pathways in order to realize the promise of social capital.

A clear and convincing theory of social capital production and of its interaction with other socio-economic dimensions is necessary in order to proceed into empirical analysis. Any empirical analysis requires assumptions and its results are only as valid as these assumptions, and the ability to make credible assumptions depends on the availability of a sound theory. Nevertheless, whatever the stage reached in the comprehension of a phenomenon, the empirical analysis allows hypotheses and predictions of the theory to be tested and provides feedback, which stimulates further progress.

The current empirical evidence suggests that a causal beneficial effect of social capital on individual health is quite strong. However, the credibility of these results depends on hypotheses about what determines individual and/or community social capital and how social capital interacts with education, employment, income, and even well-being and happiness. The circular relationship between social capital and health that has been suggested by several contributions implies that the mechanisms of social capital accumulation are more complex than previously thought and that future theoretical models should take this feature into account.

While the researcher is allowed to abstract one or a few relationships from the context and assume a particular causal path between two variables in theoretical work, this is not possible in empirical analysis. Instead, the empirical researcher must find appropriate settings or procedures to keep the complexity of the real world under control, which is a major challenge whose success depends on more or less stringent assumptions. For this reason empirical research is often subject to criticism. Controlling whatever is outside the relationship under scrutiny is the task of the identification of the structural parameters,[1] the heart of the empirical analysis. Traditional econometrics provides some useful tools with which to achieve identification, a number of which are discussed in this book. The most recent contributions achieve identification of the effect of social capital on health by adopting a technique known as instrumental variables (IV). However, the validity of these contributions rests on strong hypotheses. The large majority of early analysis looked at correlations or associations between social capital and health. Estimating associations requires fewer assumptions and might provide indications about the structural parameters, but it does not usually achieve identification. For this reason, correlations could be misleading and might lead to incorrect conclusions.

In the most recent literature in empirical economics, a great emphasis has been laid on so-called natural experiments, situations that have occurred in the real world, sometimes very localized, where exogenous and unexpected shocks randomly hit some individuals and spare others. When these shocks induce variations in one dimension of interest and leave all other dimensions unchanged, the ideal conditions that would exist only in an imaginary "social laboratory" are reproduced, and identification is easily obtained. The quest for natural experiments also promises significant advances in the empirical analysis on social capital and health.

Theory Contributions

Chapter 2, "What Is Social Capital and How Does It Work to Improve Health?" by Sherman Folland, examines the history of social capital literature in order to explain

---

[1]The structural parameters describe, for instance, how social capital influences health if all other determinants of health that are observable or unobservable to the researcher remain constant. The latter is the *ceteris paribus* hypothesis.

the sources of the current, somewhat heterogeneous definition of the phrase. It also explains the given theory of the pathways by which social capital may affect health.

Chapter 3, "How Do We Invest in Social Capital? An Exploration of an Economic Model of Social Capital and Health," by Sherman Folland, Oddvar Kaarbøe, and Kamrul Islam, begins with a utility maximization model with two variables and one constraint before expanding to a three-variable version. Social capital is described here as a form of leisure choice, which implies that it entails an opportunity cost, while investment refers to any exogenous public development that increases the marginal utility of social activity.

Chapter 4, "Social Capital: An Economic Perspective," by Audrey Laporte develops the social capital concepts and devises a dynamic model of social capital and health.

In Chapter 5, Sherman Folland and Tor Iversen discuss "How Does Social Capital Arise in Populations?" drawing on the literature to describe and explain pieces of theory on how social capital relates to age, marriage and cohabiting, culture, gender, education, and income inequality.

Empirical Contributions

Empirical analysis on the link between social capital and health requires a good deal of care and attention. The main issue to be considered is the endogeneity of social capital. The purpose of this section of the book is to provide a guide for readers on the problems frequently encountered by the researchers working in this field, enriched by several applications and a chapter devoted to the policy implications.

Chapter 6, "Measures of Social Capital" by Richard M. Scheffler and Yumna Bahgat, overviews a number of conceptual definitions of social capital and discusses perhaps the best-known and most frequently criticized characteristic of social capital, its being multifaceted. The chapter also provides a critical description of the most frequently used empirical indicators of social capital and uses the World Values Survey to describe how social capital is distributed across countries.

Chapter 7, "The Empirics of Social Capital and Health" by Lorenzo Rocco and Elena Fumagalli, discusses the econometrics of social capital and health in the context of the health reduced-form model. In particular, it analyzes the problems of endogeneity that are due to reversed causation, omitted variables, and measurement errors, as well as other econometric problems associated with the simultaneous inclusion of individual and community social capital in the same regression. The chapter also summarizes the key aspects of the peer effects model and how peer effects might interact with social capital. An extensive and detailed review with a focus on the empirics of each contribution is provided to help familiarize the reader with the empirical literature along with a discussion of how the social capital measures commonly adopted in the literature relate to experimental data. The chapter concludes with a Monte Carlo simulation to illustrate the magnitude of the bias that arises when the endogeneity of social capital is not properly addressed. A number of useful datasets reporting data on both social capital and health, most of them freely available, are schematically described in the Appendix.

Chapter 8, "Social Capital and Health in Low- and Middle-Income Countries" by José Anchorena, Lucas Ronconi, and Sachiko Ozawa, asks whether the positive correlation between social capital and health observed in high-income countries also holds in low- and middle-income countries. To answer this question, the chapter reviews the empirical literature on social capital and health in developing countries, and estimates and compares associations between social capital and health for a number of developing and developed countries using a homogenous international dataset, the International Social Survey Programme (ISSP). Some results for more and less developed regions of Argentina are also presented and discussed.

In Chapter 9, "Social Capital and Smoking," Lorenzo Rocco and Beatrice d'Hombres make a step beyond the health reduced form model to test a specific pathway previously hypothesized in the literature through which social capital influences health. This analysis tests whether social capital magnifies the impact on smoking prevalence and intensity of smoking bans in public places. A quasi-experimental setting is exploited to suggest new possibilities for the empirical work on social capital and health.

Finally, grounded in the empirical literature, Chapter 10, "Policy Implications" by Eline Aas, discusses the policy implications that could be derived from the empirical findings. It suggests a number of measures that governments could take in order to include investments in social capital in their health policies. Each chapter has benefitted from the comments of other authors, so the preparation of this work has been a valuable opportunity to build social capital among us.

References

Akerlof, G. A. 1998. Men without children. *The Economic Journal*, 115: 715–753.

Arrow, K. 1975. Gifts and exchanges. In *Altruism, Morality and Economic Theory*, ed. Phelps, E.S., New York: Russell Sage Foundation.

Becker, G. S. and Murphy, K. M. 2000. *Social Economics. Market Behavior in a Social Environment*, Cambridge, MA: The Belknap Press of Harvard University Press.

Bourdieu, P. 1985. The forms of capital. In *Handbook of Theory and Research in the Sociology of Education*, ed. Richardson, J., New York: Greenwood Publishing Group, pp. 241–258.

Coleman, J. S. 1990. *Foundations of Social Theory*, Cambridge, MA: Harvard University Press.

Durlauf, S. N. 2002. On the empirics of social capital. *The Economic Journal*, 112: F-439–479.

Glaeser, E. L., Laibson, D. and Sacerdote, B. 2002. An economic approach to social capital. *The Economic Journal*, 112: 437–458.

Kawachi, I. 1999. Social capital and community effects in population and individual health. *Annals of the New York Academy of Sciences*, 896: 120–130.

Loury, G. 1977. A dynamic theory of racial income differences. In *Women, Minorities and Employment Discrimination*, ed. LeMund, W. P., Lexington, KY: Lexington Books.

Putnam, R. D. 1995. Bowling alone: America's declining social capital. *Journal of Democracy*, 6: 65–78.

Putnam, R. D., 2000. *Bowling Alone: The Collapse and Revival of American Community*, New York: Simon & Schuster.

Putnam, R. D., Leonardi, R. and Nanetti, R. 1993. *Making Democracy Work: Civic Tradition in Modern Italy*, Princeton, NJ: Princeton University Press.

Chapter 2

What is Social Capital and How Does It Work to Improve Health?

Sherman Folland

Social capital, a recent important reconceptualization of an old and well-respected idea, developed from ideas of community known for hundreds of years — perhaps millennia. John Locke explained its value: "God having made Man such a Creature, that, in his own Judgment, it was not good for him to be alone, put him under strong Objectives of Necessity, Convenience and Inclination to drive him into Society as well as fitted him with the Understanding and Language to continue to enjoy it" (1689, p. 318).

The evidence that the social side of life is associated with specific and measurable benefits, such as better health, continues to grow. Why does this happen, via what pathways does it arrive, and what does it mean for social well-being? This chapter presents social capital theory derived from the interdisciplinary ideas that, though less formally than is typical of economic models, provides the theoretical basis on which economists can build. To add value, economics must show that economic theory provides a clear and thorough understanding of how social capital works. For example, we know that trust within a community, the size of social networks, and education benefit health, but we also wish to explain how these elements fit together and what consequences they have. In order to describe good policy, we must understand the mechanism — that is, how social capital could be enhanced to a degree that did not occur before.

To build an economic model of social capital, we benefit by first examining the noneconomic contributions from epidemiology, political science, sociology, medicine, and interdisciplinary sciences. These fields have asked important questions: What is social capital? How does it improve our health?

9

The meaning of *social capital* depends on how it is used. Glenn Loury (1977), a forerunner in the study of social capital, showed that traditional economic analysis could not well explain the roots of income differences between blacks and whites. Loury identified the missing element as social capital, which he defined as the influences of family and community on the individual.

The sociologist James Coleman developed a theory of social capital, identifying it in three parts: "Obligations and expectations, information channels, and social norms." (These categories, in the main, survive in present-day social capital writing.) Coleman argued that the categories apply "both within the family and in the community outside" (Coleman, 1988, p. 895).

Pierre Bourdieu (1985) described social capital as the benefit of a network of friends and acquaintances and of membership in a group, which might be family, a social group, or other institutions, such as a tribe or a political party, that adheres to the individual agent like a "credential." We also find in Bourdieu a theory of the relationship of social capital to other forms of capital.

Robert Putnam, who ranks as the best known and most widely read of present-day social capital researchers, described the beneficial characteristics of relationships, groups, networks, and social norms experienced by individuals and community as trust, honesty, volunteerism, sociability, and engagement in community affairs (1993, p. 291). Putnam applied these characteristics in his empirical work, elements of which have been widely adopted by others.

Is social capital an economic concept like other economic capital? Leading economic theorists Kenneth Arrow and James Tobin objected to this usage (Robison *et al.*, 2002), contending that capital requires one to forego current benefits for future benefits, producing capital entails opportunity costs. Does maintaining family, networks of friends, and ties to the community have opportunity costs? Does it require "investing" now so as to gain future benefit? It is clear now that social capital often fits this picture, because its cost can be measured in time spent, if not also in money, and because individuals often invest time in social relationships in the expectation of future benefits. However, some elements of social capital, like social norms, seem thrust upon us, perhaps even without our awareness. Given these considerations, one can agree that social capital, while not a physical capital, is a form of economic capital much like the well-recognized concept of like human capital.

The term *social capital* elicits the intended idea of a social tissue or glue that the research community commonly understands. Social capital is durable, as is evident in time series data: It depreciates and must be replenished (invested in) in order to be maintained, and empirical studies have indicated periods of decline. As a practical matter, social capital is clear to a substantial and growing research community, which understands the term and has no difficulty designing clearly focused studies based on it.

Two additional concepts help to identify distinctions in social relationships: *bridging* and *bonding*. As Putnam (2000) observed, some social groups engage and reinforce the identities of like people, such as church groups and ethnic fraternities. These inward-looking groups are *bonding* groups. In contrast, *bridging* groups are those whose members reach out beyond themselves in order to link to assets outside the group and encourage the diffusion of information.

Does the family count as social capital? Loury (1977), Coleman (1988), and Putnam (2000), early theorizers on the subject, identified family as an important influence on the social glue, yet many researchers insisted later that social capital is strictly a community concept. In the past decade, econometric studies have often tended to separate marital status and family characteristics from the "social capital" variables. Many of these studies are ecological, comparing the mean characteristics of geographic areas, such as countries, states, and cities. However, the concept of "individual social capital" is increasingly studied, and this category tends to perform better in econometric analyses in which both individual and community social capital variables appear. Certainly, it seems more natural now to include family as an element of individual social capital. While Putnam once stated that "the family is the most fundamental form of social capital" (1995, p. 65), there is no need to force the issue; when econometric research separates family variables from the social capital set, the family variables are inevitably included as covariate variables.

Understood as family, extended family, friends, and community or social network, social capital influences our lives and provides an important social glue, a necessary element of our existence. How does it affect one's health? The literature offers four plausible explanations. First, relationships can ease stress. Biologists and medical scientists corroborate that stress can result in ill health (e.g., Sapolsky, 1998). Psychological health benefits from the right blend of social company and time alone. Even though some relationships are stressful, the overwhelming predominance of human behavior suggests that social contacts are generally beneficial. This pathway for benefits to health, however, suggests many deeper issues that may be mined in future research. Some examples: Is some basic level of stress tonic for humans, an interior solution? Can the level of stress in populations be quantified? Are sociability and stress inversely correlated empirically?

Second, one's network of friends, relatives, and acquaintances provide a potentially rich source of information. Information provides guidance on healthful personal behaviors as well as news about the availability of medical treatments and the symptoms that they can alleviate. Friends are a common source of recommendations to physicians. When a spouse or friend cajoles you to exercise or to quit smoking, that too, is information.

Third, family, friends, and community add value to one's life, which alters the rate of tradeoff one chooses between the pleasures of "health bads" like smoking and the risks of illness or death (Folland, 2008). A related effect is the increased sense of responsibility one feels toward one's relationships and oneself. For example, a new father may decide to take better care of his own health once he is responsible for the long-term well-being and growth of his child.

Fourth, Jennifer Mellor (2005) suggests that a social network can provide the basis for a group organization developed to improve the healthful conditions of the community (see also Kawachi *et al.,* 1997).

Summary and Concluding Remarks

Covariate variables, those intended to control for confounding effects, include many that are also associated with the production of social capital. These variables help to determine the setting for the econometric work, but the relationships among them are complex and may not yet be fully understood. Several such variables are developed in depth in Chapter 5, entitled "How Does Social Capital Arise in Populations?"

Gender: Men's and women's patterns of communication, risk aversion, and, when small children are involved, the sense of responsibility differ, suggesting that there also may be a different patterns of responsibility to one's own health.

Mobility: Glaeser, Laibson and Sacerdote (2002) found that moving residence locations tends to reduce one's set of friends and acquaintances, which could reduce one's health.

Education: Education is positively related to health. Perhaps the intelligence education generates provides the individual with health information, but an older argument points out that people who invest in education tend to make plans with longer time horizons and correspondingly lower discount rates for future returns, so they may put more value on their future health. Empirical tests designed to discriminate between these two hypotheses tended to find education to be the active causal factor (Lleras-Muney, 2005).

Income and Income Inequality: We know that very low incomes, such as those that exist in the developing world, are contributors to poor health (Pritchett and Summers, 1996). In developed countries the income/health relationship is more difficult. Deaton and Paxson (2001) find no relationship between income and health once incomes rise above a middling level. Income inequality poses a different problem, as relative poverty may generate its own unhealthful stress. Wilkinson and Pickett (2006) found in a meta-analysis that greater income inequality is most often associated with poorer population health. Kawachi and Kennedy (1999) reasoned that income inequality may mean that segments of society do not communicate well across income barriers, so they lack the ability to develop social capital.

Insurance: Health insurance enables one to afford treatment for costly, life-threatening medical surprises. Insurance also increases one's consumption of health care, a clear result of the RAND Health Insurance Experiment (RHIE) (Newhouse, 1993). While the RHIE reported that the extra health care had little or no effect on health status, Gruber (2008) found that the RHIE subjects were not wholly uninsured but that they had coverage after a deductible of $1,000. Other studies (Carrie and Gruber, 1997; Hanratty, 1996; Doyle, 2005) found that the lack of health insurance or the lapse of Medicaid coverage has significant effects on health measures, including mortality rates.

Health Care: Despite earlier skepticism, health care availability in populations not only improves health but is cost-effective. Murphy and Topel (2005) found that gains in life expectancy from 1970 to 2000 were worth several trillion dollars, far more than we spent on medical research. Cutler (2004) estimates that nearly half of life expectancy gains between 1950 and 2000 were due to medical advances.

Lifestyle: Many Americans have undertaken unhealthful behaviors, such as smoking, lack of exercise, and overeating, that are detrimental to health. With the exception of smoking, these behaviors stand out so much in American statistics that they alone can account for Americans' deficiencies in international comparisons of life expectancy (Comanor, Frech, and Miller, 2006).

The next three chapters extend received theory. Chapter 3, "How Do We Invest in Social Capital? An Exploration of an Economic Model of Social Capital and Health," develops the analytics of a case in which choice variables include social capital and goods, which have effects either beneficial or harmful to health. Investment is made exogenously through social capital enabling factors. Chapter 4, "Social Capital: An Economic Perspective," develops social capital concepts and constructs a dynamic model which features time patterns of both health and of social capital. Chapter 5, "How Does Social Capital Arise in Populations?" develops and explains theoretical and empirically related literature on the effects of age, marriage, culture, gender, income, and education on social capital and health.

References

Bourdieu, P. 1985. The form of capital. In *Handbook of Theory and Research in Sociology*, ed. Richardson, J., New York: Greenwood, pp. 241–258.

Coleman, J. 1988. Social capital in the creation of human capital. *The American Journal of Sociology*, Supplement, 94: S95–S120.

Comanor, W. S., Frech, H. E. and Miller, R. 2006. Is the United States an outlier in health care and health outcomes? A preliminary analysis. *International Journal of Health Care Finance and Economics*, 6: S95–S120.

Currie, J. and Gruber, J. 1996. Saving babies: The efficiency and cost of recent changes in Medicaid eligibility of pregnant women. *Journal of Political Economy*, 106: 1263–1296.

Deaton, A. and Paxson, C. 2001. Mortality, education, income and inequality among American cohorts. In *Themes in the Economics of Aging*, ed. Wise, D., Chicago: Chicago University Press, pp. 129–170.

Doyle, J. 2005. Health insurance, treatment and outcomes: Using auto accidents as health shocks. *The Review of Economics and Statistics*, 87: 256–270.

Folland, S. 2008. An economic model of social capital and health. *Health Economics, Policy and Law*, 3: 1–15.

Glaeser, E. L., Laibson, D. and Sacerdote, B. 2002. An economic approach to social capital. *The Economic Journal*, 112: F437–F458.

Gruber, J. 2008. Covering the uninsured in the United States. *Journal of Economic Literature*, 46: 571–606.

Hanratty, M. 1996. Canadian national health insurance. *The American Economic Review*, 86: 276–284.

Kawachi, I. 1999. Social capital and community effects in population and individual health. *Annals of the New York Academy of Sciences*, 896: 120–130.

Kawachi, I. and Kennedy, B. P. 1999. Income inequality and health: Pathways and mechanics. *Health Services Research*, 34: 215–227.

Kawachi, I. *et al.* 1997. Social capital income inequality and mortality. *American Journal of Public Health*, 87: 1491–1498.

Lleras-Muney, A. 2005. The relationship between education and adult mortality in the United States. *Review of Economic Studies*, 72: 189–221.

Locke, J. (orig. pub. 1689) 1960. *Two Treatises on Government*, Cambridge: Cambridge University Press.

Loury, G. 1977. A dynamic theory of racial differences. In *Women, Minorities and Employment Discrimination*, eds. Wallace, P. B. and LaMond, A., Lexington, MA: Lexington Books.

Mellor, J. M. and Milyo, J. 2005. State social capital and individual health status. *Journal of Health Policy Politics & Law*, 30: 1101–1130.

Newhouse, J. P. 1993. *Free For All? Lessons from the RAND Health Insurance Experiment*, Cambridge, MA: Harvard University Press.

Pritchett, L. and Summers, L. 1996. Wealthier is healthier. *Journal of Human Resources*, 25: 841–868.

Putnam, R. D. 1993. *Making Democracy Work*, Princeton, NJ: Princeton University Press.

Putnam, R. D. 1995. Bowling alone: American declining social capital. *Journal of Democracy*, 6: 65–78.

Putnam, R. D. 2000. *Bowling Alone:The Collapse and Revival of American Community*, New York: Simon and Schuster.

Robison, L., Schmid, A. A. and Siles, M. 2002. Is social capital really capital? *Review of Social Economy*, 60: 1–21.

Sapolsky, R. M. 1998. *Why Zebras Don't Get Ulcers: An Updated Guide to Stress Related Diseases and Coping*, New York: W. H. Freeman and Company.

Wilkinson, R. G. and Pickett, K. E. 2006. Income inequality and population health: A review of explanations of the evidence. *Social Science & Medicine*, 62: 1768–1784.

Chapter 3

How Do We Invest in Social Capital? An Exploration of an Economic Model of Social Capital and Health

Sherman Folland, Oddvar Kaarbøe and Kamrul Islam

Economic research on social capital usually finds that increments of social interaction improve health. Urban economists and planners naturally seek public projects that encourage residents to interact beneficially. Many such projects, such as public parks and playgrounds, beaches, policing and safety, local transportation, and improvements in shopping areas, can be expensive but it is likely that the city dweller tends to consider the expense only in general terms when voting whether to approve a tax increase. For this reason our approach here takes the insertion of such public goods as exogenous to the choice of the individual subject, maximizing his or her utility.

Social capital, which might best be measured as one's network of personal bonds, is not constituted of the public projects themselves but is enabled by them. The choice of social interaction entails opportunity costs, largely in time and wages lost, that are not usually incorporated into the social capital literature, so their possible consequences remain to be explored. This approach reveals the many interactions between such public projects, social capital, and the rest of the market economy. Somewhat oversimplified effects, such as "membership in a social club improves one's health," have often been hypothesized, but even a two-variable model with one budget constraint reveals more realistic complications. A more extensive three-variable model illustrates that the interactions grow at an almost geometric rate as one adds more variables.

The usefulness of working through a utility-maximization model of social capital and health lies in its ability to test the consistency of our facts and common assumptions. We can examine its implications in order to improve our understanding of our empirical work.

The Environment of the Model

We assume that a public-good investment, E, represents an enabler of social capital, S, if it enhances the marginal utility of S that the subject enjoys from social activities. The public good may provide utility independent of S, but more importantly, it enhances the pleasure of social interaction. We introduce three kinds of *other goods*, each sequentially called C: A composite good that neither adds nor subtracts from the utility of S; a health "good" like health care that improves health on the margin, although it may or may not be complementary to the project; and a health "bad," cigarette consumption, that is enjoyable and adds to utility but harms health and the survival probability. Finally, we would like to look into the relationship between education and social capital. In this case, let the other good represent education increments that are costly. We are specifically interested in whether a public subsidy for education could — as a side benefit — increase social capital

We begin by examining utility maximization with two variables, S and C, and one budget constraint. Utility $= U(S, E, C)$. Let S absorb all leisure time during a period of 24 hours. Here, a "day" is a metaphor for the subject's working life, hence the model includes no lifecycle features. Let γ represent the probability that the subject will survive the day. Since the day is uniform throughout, the expected utility is identical to the portion of the subject's working life that he or she can expect to enjoy. The individual's budget constraint is $w(24 - S) \geq pC$, where w is the wage and p is the price of C. This approach treats all non-work time as social capital. Since we view social capital to include interactions within the family, as did the early writers (see Chapter 2), the assumption is not so extreme as it may seem at first. It also simplifies the exposition.

A Bare-Bones Model

Let C at price p represents the only use of income (a two-good model), and S activities which absorb all leisure time, making it identical to leisure hours. The standard labor/leisure model serves as a useful starting point. In Figure 3.1, the line segment AB represents the tradeoff curve, with a slope of $-w/p$. The equilibrium shown at H_1 implies that $-U_S/U_C = -w/p$. It follows that, if the marginal utility of S is enhanced by the social capital-enabling project, then $-U_S/U_C > -{'}U_S/U_C$,

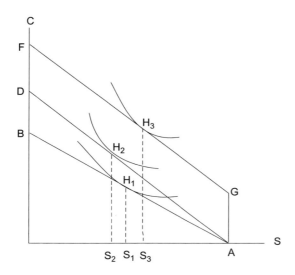

Figure 3.1: A labor/social capital tradeoff.

where 'U_S is the new marginal utility of S, so that a new equilibrium will arise somewhere to the southeast of H_1, indicating a greater demand for social capital.

A higher wage gives the tradeoff curve of line segment AD, leading to a lower equilibrium value of social capital at H_2 because there is now a higher monetary incentive to work. In conventional theory, there may eventually be a backward-bending portion of the labor supply curve, not shown, derived from successive changes in the wage. A literal interpretation of such a pattern would be that one turns to more social time when one becomes satisfied with one's income, but this interpretation would be too literal and would ignore the interactions of wage effects with other variables, as we develop in a later section. What is clear is that real wage increases change the relative price of social capital and the other good, providing the incentive to move away from S.

Finally, if the subject gets additional money sufficient to buy AG, the tradeoff curve becomes line segment GF, which induces an equilibrium with greater levels of both S and C, provided they are normal goods.

A Model Incorporating the Social Capital and Health Hypothesis

There are two limitations of using the labor/leisure model (Figure 3.1) in our context: It does not include the hypothesized health effects, so it does not tell the full social capital story, and completing the model with health effects shows it to be substantially different in terms of qualitative implications. Consider a version in which the subject maximizes expected utility with the risks to survival, which depend on health:

$$\text{LaGrangian Function}: L = \gamma U(S, E, C) + \varphi[w(24 - S) - pC] \qquad (3.1)$$

where the survival probability, $\gamma = f(Health)$, and $Health = h(S, C)$. To minimize non-essential complexity, let γ be linear in S and C so that $\frac{\partial \gamma}{\partial S} > 0$, $\frac{\partial^2 \gamma}{\partial S, S} = 0$, $\frac{\partial^2 \gamma}{\partial C, C} = 0$. The first derivative effects of C on γ, which depend on the definition of C, are explained later.

As before, γ is the survival probability; S is social capital; E is the public good; C is the *other good* which we treat sequentially as a composite consumer good, a healthcare good, and the health bad cigarette consumption; w is the wage; and p is the price of C. This construction implies no utility after death.[2]

Since E is exogenous, the model becomes a familiar model of two variables and one constraint. Its first-order conditions are:

$$L_S = \gamma_S U(\cdot) + \gamma U_S - w\varphi = 0 \qquad (3.2)$$

$$L_C = \gamma_C U(\cdot) + \gamma U_C - p\varphi = 0 \qquad (3.3)$$

$$L_\varphi = w(24 - S) - pC = 0 \qquad (3.4)$$

Equations (3.2) and (3.3) combine to produce a variant of the conventional efficiency condition that the ratio of net marginal utilities equals the ratio of prices.

$$\frac{\gamma_S U(\cdot) + \gamma U_S}{\gamma_C U(\cdot) + \gamma U_C} = \frac{w}{p} \qquad (3.5)$$

This model would have reduced to the labor/leisure tradeoff adaptation if we had set $\gamma \equiv 1.0$.

The structure of this two-good model and of our approach can be seen by first foreswearing knowledge about the character of the variable C. A two-good model is often sufficient to reveal the main tendencies of the subject's responses. The central questions are: (1) Does the public investment tend to increase social capital? (2) Does the investment tend to improve the subject's health? (3) Does a rise in wage raise or lower social capital or change other health-related variables?

---

[2]Post-death utility indicates that the living subject gains utility from his bequest-related plans.

For convenience, the required cross-partials are given here:

$$L_{SS} = 2\gamma_S U_S + \gamma U_{SS} \tag{3.6}$$

$$L_{CS} = \gamma_C U_S + \gamma_S U_C + \gamma U_{SC} \tag{3.7}$$

$$L_{CC} = 2\gamma_C U_C + \gamma U_{CC} \tag{3.8}$$

$$L_{\varphi S} = -w \tag{3.9}$$

$$L_{\varphi C} = -p \tag{3.10}$$

$$L_{\varphi\varphi} = 0 \tag{3.11}$$

$$L_{SE} = \gamma_S U_E + \gamma U_{SE} \tag{3.12}$$

$$L_{CE} = \gamma_C U_E + \gamma U_{CE} \tag{3.13}$$

$$L_{\varphi E} = 0 \tag{3.14}$$

Several items in these terms use a commonly assumed sign: Conventionally $U_{CC} < 0$; $U_{SS} < 0$; $U_S > 0$; $U_C > 0$. The survival effects depend on the definition of C: For common consumption goods, $\gamma_C = 0$; for health care, $\gamma_C > 0$; and for cigarettes, $\gamma_C < 0$. Cross-partials include $U_{SE} > 0$, by definition of E, and U_{CE} is more speculative, as well as dependent on the definition of C. In several cases the introduction of survival effects makes the term's sign unknown. The most difficult expression to align with typical empirical work is cigarettes. Reconsider Eq. (3.7), noting that the first two expressions contrast the harm of smoking with the benefit, and whether one's social network enhances or lowers the marginal utility of cigarettes depends on one's social group, so that $U_{SC} > ? < 0$. These terms matter in calculating qualitative effects of the investment.

Using Cramér's Rule, the solutions to $\partial C/\partial E$ and $\partial S/\partial E$ are given in Eqs. (3.15) and (3.16) with the H determinant positive:

$$\partial C/\partial E = \{w^2(\gamma_C U_E + \gamma U_{CE}) - (wp(\gamma_S U_{SE}))\}/H \quad > ? < 0 \tag{3.15}$$

and

$$\partial S/\partial E = p[p(\gamma_S U_E + \gamma U_{SE}) - w(\gamma_C U_E + \gamma U_{CE})]/H \quad > ? < 0 \tag{3.16}$$

Three Cases of an Exogenous Public Investment

Consider when several social capital investment scenarios created by conceiving the *other good*, C, are of different types. First, consumer goods, like transportation and clothing, have no apparent effect on survival probability and may not bear either a complement or substitute relationship to a social capital good, such as a new city park. In contrast, another type of good, C, could include health care, which improves health and survival. Demand at exercise centers and health care clinics that improve ambulation may be encouraged by a new park that provides athletic activities. Finally, health bads, such as cigarette consumption, while not stimulated by the public investment, may interact with other market variables through their effect on survival.

Case 1: Let $\gamma_C = 0$, $U_C > 0$, and $U_{CE} = 0$. A consumption good that is neither related to health nor to public investment. Here the planner's target, better health through greater social capital, has no competition. From Eqs. (3.15) and (3.16), $\frac{\partial S}{\partial E} > 0$ and $\frac{\partial C}{\partial E} < 0$. The subject simply shifts toward social capital. Of course, in this two-variable model C is synonymous with real income and, by design, income and social capital must move in opposite directions. This scenario is plausible to the extent that social relationships take place mainly outside of the work environment, so it includes the opportunity cost of lowered work time or effort. However, this approach may risk neglecting the significant social interaction that takes place at work. By adding one or more additional uses of income, the rigid tradeoff between S and C is relaxed.

Case 2: $\gamma_C > 0$, $U_C > 0$, and $U_{CE} \geq 0$. If the other good, C, is health care, it improves survival on the margin and may or may not be a complement to the public investment. The effect of an exogenous public investment, E, may cause this good to compete with social capital because both have a beneficial effect on survival, whether the public good is a complement for a good that provides improved survival, a substitute for such a good, or neither. Re-examining Eqs. (3.15) and (3.16), C competes with S in this scenario, so $\frac{\partial C}{\partial E} > ? < 0$ and $\frac{\partial S}{\partial E} > ? < 0$.

Case 3: $\gamma_C < 0$, $U_C > 0$, and $U_{CE} = 0$. If the other good is a health bad, like cigarettes, it would likely be unrelated to the public-investment good. Cigarette consumption provides utility, but it reduces one's survival probability. Cigarettes neither substitute nor complement a park or playground. Social capital gains doubly in this case because it provides utility but also because its competitor, C, reduces the amount of time one expects to enjoy the public good. Thus, $\frac{\partial C}{\partial E} < 0$ and $\frac{\partial S}{\partial E} > 0$.

Other Effects

Case 4: $\gamma_C = 0$. $U_C > 0$ and $U_{SC} > 0$. Let the *other good* represent education increments that are costly to the subject, such as college. Education levels correlate positively with social capital in this literature, and education is often suggested as a possible input to the production function of social capital. (See Chapter 5, "How Does Social Capital Arise in Populations?") Public policy that reduces the price of education could provide the side benefit of increasing social capital. Let the other good, C, represent college education and find the responses of S and C to the price of college as:

$$\partial S/\partial p = \{C[-p(\gamma_C U_S + \gamma_S U_C + \gamma U_{SC}) + w[(2\gamma_C U_C)$$

$$+ \gamma U_{CC}] + pw\varphi\}/H \tag{3.17}$$

$$\frac{\partial C}{\partial p} = \{C[-p((2\gamma_S U_S) + \gamma U_{SS}) + w(\gamma_C U_S + \gamma_S U_C + \gamma U_{SC})] - w^2\varphi\}/H \tag{3.18}$$

The first parenthesis in Eq. (3.17) describes the marginal utility effect of college, and this expression enters negatively, detracting from social capital. The same expression appears in (3.18) and enters as a bump to C. Both equations include ambiguities, $[(2\gamma_C U_C) + \gamma U_{CC})$ in (3.17) and $((2\gamma_S U_S) + \gamma U_{SS})$ in (3.18). In both equations the bracketed expressions adjust or partly offset the clearly signed ending expressions. Taking ending expressions the latter as the main tendencies suggests that college education declines with price, while social capital competes. In Figure 3.1, the effect of an increase in p could be illustrated by the shift from tradeoff line AD to line AB. In the bare-bones model, the increase in price causes the equilibrium to shift from H_2 to H_1, causing C to fall and S to rise, although well-behaved indifference curves could cause both to fall. The empirical question remain concerning whether the subsidy would increase both the level of college education and the level of social capital.

How a Composite Consumption Good Interacts with a Health Bad: An Exercise with Three Variables

$$\gamma_X = 0, \quad U_X > 0, \quad \gamma_C < 0, \quad \gamma_S > 0$$

To explore a three variable model, let C be a health bad, and let the new variable, X, represent the composite consumption good. Here social capital enhances the expected utility of X by extending survival, while C harms both S and X by reducing survival.

$$\text{To maximize } L = \gamma U(S, E, C, X) + \varphi(w(24 - S) - pC - X) \quad (3.19)$$

$$L_S = \gamma_S U(\cdot) + \gamma U_S - w\varphi = 0 \quad (3.20)$$

$$L_C = \gamma_C U(\cdot) + \gamma U_C - p\varphi = 0 \quad (3.21)$$

$$L_X = \gamma U_X - \varphi = 0 \quad (3.22)$$

$$L_\varphi = w(24 - S) - pC - X = 0 \quad (3.23)$$

Apply Cramér's Rule, given that the Hessian determinant is negative.

$$\partial S / \partial E = \{-p[-L_{SE}(-L_{XC} + pL_{XX}) + L_{CE}(-L_{SX} + wL_{XX})]$$
$$+ [-L_{SE}(-L_{CC} + pL_{XC}) + L_{CE}(-L_{SC} + wL_{XC})]\}/H$$
$$(3.24)$$

$$\partial C / \partial E = \{w[-L_{SE}(-L_{XC} + pL_{XX}) + L_{CE}(-L_{SX} + wL_{XX})]$$
$$+ [L_{SS}L_{CE} - L_{SC}L_{SE} + L_{XS}(pL_{SE} - wL_{CE})]\}/H$$
$$(3.25)$$

Compare the qualitative results with those in Case 3, where demand for the health bad was reduced in favor of increased social capital. The addition of X introduces ambiguity in the effects of E on S and C. To demonstrate, apply the terms from Eqs. (3.6) through (3.14) and the interactions with the new variable X. (These are brought together in the Appendix to this chapter.) As a result, we have:

$$L_{SE} > 0, \quad L_{CX} < 0, \quad L_{XX} < 0, \quad L_{CE} < 0,$$
$$L_{SX} > 0, \quad L_{CC} < 0, \quad L_{CS}, > ? < \quad L_{SS} > ? <$$

In (3.24) the first bracketed expression is positive, contributes to an increase in S, similar to the Case 3 result.[3] Cross-partials like L_{XC}, L_{SC}, and L_{SS} are essential to the story and cannot be ignored, as they introduce ambiguities.

A similar conclusion is found in (3.25). The first bracketed expression is positive, contributing to a reduction in demand for cigarettes, but the remainder of Eq. 3.25 introduces questions. Such questions are often introduced because of

---

[3]The expression $(-L_{XC} - pL_{XX}) < 0$ satisfies the second-order condition for the bordered Hessians.

survival effects. For example, $L_{SS} = 2\gamma_S U_S + U_{SS} > ? < 0$. The concavity of the utility function implies that $U_{SS} < 0$, yet the troublesome survival effects leave uncertain the sign of L_{SS}. The health effects of social capital constitute the main point and cannot be discarded. Consider also $L_{SC} = \gamma_S U_C + \gamma_C U_S + U_{SC} > ? < 0$. It may be "unhealthy" to include a term like $\gamma_S U_C$ as it suggests that a benefit of social capital is to extend the number of hours you can enjoy your cigarettes. While this result seems odd, if we are to take the individual's utility seriously, it cannot be dismissed.

Summary and Concluding Remarks

In many cultures most social activity takes place outside the workplace. When the boundary line between work and leisure is flexible, social capital will compete with the income with which to buy market goods. By treating all leisure time as devoted to social activities in these models, we see that the conventional labor/leisure tradeoff model describes the underlying fundamentals but that it is limited in that its implications differ substantially from our understanding and in that it does not tell the story of the effect of social capital on health. To explore these ideas we presented two expected utility maximization models in which increments of social capital improve the probability of survival.

The two-variable models make the main tendencies clear. Here social capital is an endogenous choice variable. To observe the effects of changes in the variable, we introduce an exogenous public investment, such as a park, a playground, or an enhanced level of safety, that enhances the marginal utility of social capital. The public investment's effects depend on the nature of the *other good*.

When the other good, such as clothing, transportation, food, or housing, brings utility but provides no effect on health, the public investment stimulates greater demand for social capital. When the other good, such as gyms or health clinics, also improves survival, then the two goods compete. When the other good is a health bad, such as cigarettes, then the demand for social capital increases. Finally, when we artificially reduce the price of higher education, the most likely result is an increase in education but it may include a reduction in social capital, however this last result depends on the marginal product of education in the production function of social capital.

As expected, an expansion of the model to three variables introduces new ambiguities, even in the health bad case, which one would think to be the simplest and clearest. At the most general level, the models suggest that, when social capital has opportunity costs, and public investments intended to enable social capital may bring both benefits and some unintended consequences.

Appendix

$$L_{CX} = \gamma_C U_X + \gamma U_{XX} \tag{3.26}$$

$$L_{XX} = \gamma U_{XX} \tag{3.27}$$

$$L_{SX} = \gamma_S U_X + \gamma U_{SX} \tag{3.28}$$

$$L_{SS} = 2\gamma_S U_S + \gamma U_{SS} \tag{3.29}$$

$$L_{CS} = \gamma_C U_S + \gamma_S U_C + \gamma U_{SC} \tag{3.30}$$

$$L_{CC} = 2\gamma_C U_C + \gamma U_{CC} \tag{3.31}$$

$$L_{\varphi S} = -w \tag{3.32}$$

$$L_{\varphi C} = -p \tag{3.33}$$

$$L_{\varphi \varphi} = 0 \tag{3.34}$$

$$L_{SE} = \gamma_S U_E + \gamma U_{SE} \tag{3.35}$$

$$L_{CE} = \gamma_C U_E + \gamma U_{CE} \tag{3.36}$$

$$L_{\varphi E} = 0 \tag{3.37}$$

Chapter 4

Social Capital: An Economic Perspective

Audrey Laporte

The literature on social capital and health is large and growing but amorphous. An outside observer would have the impression that social capital is an important factor in population health but would be hard pressed from reading the literature to say exactly what social capital is, much less how it works. If that observer were restricted to particular subsets of the literature, he or she would find that researchers who work in one subset have well-defined notions of social capital but those who work in another subset also have a well-defined concept of social capital that may bear no resemblance at all to that of researchers in other subsets. Makers of health policy who wish to derive the greatest value from the academic literature on social capital broadly defined will need a taxonomy.

Taxonomies tend to be discipline-specific, so this chapter provides a taxonomy from the perspective of standard health economic theory. Readers from other disciplines may well disagree with how we have defined social capital, but we hope that they will feel inspired to produce taxonomies of their own. From the economist's perspective the keyword in the term *social capital* is *capital*. Arrow (2000) and Solow (2000) both observed that the term *capital* is often used in a different sense from how economists typically use it. In much of the social capital literature, the term *capital* is taken to indicate the presence of a stock of something, without much attention given to where that stock came from. In other areas of economics, the process by which such a stock is accumulated and de-cumulated is fundamental to the analysis. Economists have a well-defined notion of capital as a durable stock that can be accumulated through investment activities that produce ultimate outputs — in this case, health. Such stock can be depleted as a consequence of its being used as a productive input, and it may depreciate simply as the result of the passage of time, even if it is not used. Some strands of the social capital literature have this concept of *capital* in mind, whereas others use the term *social capital* to cover a range of publicly provided goods, and still others use the term as a construct along the lines of what economists refer to as a public good, which (confusingly enough) is different from the concept of publicly provided goods. The purpose of this chapter is, to then provide an economist's characterization of some of the most important sub-categories of social capital with the aim of encouraging economists to work in the field and giving researchers from other disciplines some notion of how economists tend to think about social capital.

Broad Types of Social Capital

It is probably fair to say that the first type of social capital to enter the health literature was a type that we would regard as a form of public good (Wilkinson, 1996). To economists the term *public good* has a particular — some would say peculiar — meaning. Classic public goods are "non-rivalrous" and "non-excludable." Non-excludable public goods are those from which everyone in the community benefits by dint of living in the community and from which no one can be excluded by, say, the requirement to pay a price for access. Non-rivalrous public goods are those whose benefit to a member of the community is not reduced by the fact that another member of the community benefits from it. Such non-excludable, non-rivalrous public goods are like radio broadcasts: Anyone can receive them, and the fact that one person plucks the signal out of the airwaves does not reduce the strength of the signal someone else can pluck from the airwaves. This branch of the social capital literature tends to deal with the effects of the characteristics of a society as a whole. Perhaps the most familiar example of this strand of literature relates to the impact of income inequality on health, where income inequality reflects the degree of social cohesion. Seen from the perspective of social capital, in the income inequality literature the key fact is not that some people are poor in an absolute sense but the impact of inequality. In other words, the fact that poverty tends to go along with poor health is not denied by this literature, but the focus is the impact of inequality as an independent determinant of health. An increase in inequality, even one that did not leave the bottom end of the income distribution any worse off in real terms, would still be expected to reduce the amount of that community's social capital and, therefore, to have a negative impact on population health. Even controlling for absolute poverty, in this strand of the literature increasing inequality would be regarded as a form of public bad: A type of social pollution. Its individual impact may depend on where one happens to be in the income distribution, but it is presumed to have a negative impact on everyone. While it may be possible to develop community policies aimed at the community's level of social capital, social capital is strictly exogenous to the individual. Bill Gates or Warren Buffet might be able to affect it through individual activities, but the vast majority of us cannot.

Another important strand of the literature characterizes social capital as a form of publicly provided private good that is either free or heavily subsidized. The Petris Index developed by Richard Scheffler and colleagues at UC Berkeley could be classed here (see e.g., Brown and Scheffler, 2006). The Petris Index measures the supply-side of community social capital by calculating the percentage of people employed in religious or community-based organizations in a defined geographic area. In economic terms, this type of social capital is a mechanism for allocating resources to individuals. Unlike the pure public form, it is both rivalrous and excludable, as it does not freely radiate across the community but must be rationed by some mechanism or another. That mechanism may (and should) involve allocating it to individuals who will most benefit from it, but its rivalrous nature means that the more one person gets, the less someone else gets. Moreover, this type of social capital (e.g., meals-on-wheels services) may be offered in the community, but whether an individual is eligible for these services and how much they receive is beyond their immediate control. The degree to which this sort of social capital is available in any part of the community may well reflect the degree of social cohesion in that community, but its mechanism of operation differs from the pure public good case.

The final category of social capital comes closest to the economist's notion of a capital good: Individual social capital is a form of social capital that requires the individual to make investments in building and maintaining it. It is similar to the economist's notion of human capital (e.g., education, skills acquisition), but it involves participating in a social contract. In terms of the health literature, research that focuses on the health effects of the networks to which individuals belong fall under this heading of social capital research. Here, the individual has control and invests in his or her social capital by, for example, building social networks through participation in clubs, sports, church, and community groups. Participation in these types of activities can be viewed as a form of non-market insurance; by contributing their efforts when they can, individuals earn the right to draw on the network when they need help. Perhaps the most familiar examples of research into this type of social capital are by Putnam (2000) and Folland (2008).

The focus of this chapter is on modeling the type of social capital in which an individual can make investments, since this area of research is underdeveloped. While we mention some of the interactions among the other types of social capital, our focus is on a model of investment in individual social capital. We leave the development of a more detailed model that involves all three types of social capital to future research.

Theoretical Framework

We begin with a model that builds on the standard Grossman (1972) investment in the health capital framework. The Grossman framework is an appropriate starting point for several. First, it recognizes that health deteriorates with age and that individuals must invest in their health in order to affect this rate of decline. It also incorporates the fact that individuals' decisions about investments in their health (through consumption of medical care, exercise, etc.) in past periods of their life have implications for their future health statuses. Further, using the Grossman framework allows us to investigate how adding concepts of social capital to the standard model affects its predictions about individual health-related behavior. The Grossman framework looks at individuals' health-related decisions from a lifetime perspective, so it yields predictions about trajectories of health and health-related behaviors through the entire lifespan. Therefore, the individual in the Grossman model is forward-looking; he or she may make mistakes in expectations about the future and may have to modify decisions as a result of unexpected changes in exogenous variables or circumstances generally, but this framework allows us to treat the individual as taking account of future consequences of current decisions. This is why the Grossman model is referred to as a model of investment in health capital and is why it is a suitable framework in which to incorporate individual decisions about investment in individual social capital and how that social capital may affect the individual's health.

Consider an optimization problem in which the individual aims to maximize her lifetime utility (U) from period $t = 0$ to t, subject to a series of constraints. The individual's per period utility function is given by:

$$U(C_t, H_t, L_t) \tag{4.1}$$

The individual's utility in each period t depends on consumption (C_t) that takes place during period t, of her stock of health capital (H_t) at the beginning of period t, which will depend on what she did in the past and on leisure (L_t). All of these elements (C_t, H_t, and L_t) have a positive impact on the individual's utility so that her marginal utility with respect to each is positive, that is, U_C, U_H, and $U_L > 0$ but declining (i.e., U_{CC}, U_{HH}, $U_{LL} < 0$).

The individual aims to maximize her lifetime utility but must do so within certain constraints. A key aspect of the inter-temporal nature of the problem lies in the fact that the value of H in period t depends on previous decisions. H in this model is health capital, which refers not so much to how the individual might be feeling on any particular day but to her state of healthfulness broadly defined. It is a durable good in the sense that the individual's health in period $t + 1$ depends not just on her current health-related actions but on her state of health in period t. We mentioned above that health in period t depends on the whole sequence of health-related actions undertaken in past periods. We can represent these decisions by H_{t-1}, which is the individual stock of health in period $t - 1$. Bringing these notions together, we write an "equation of motion" for health capital. We work in this model in discrete time terms, so we have to make explicit decisions about whether actions undertaken in period t affect health in period t or, operating with a one-period lag, affect health in period $t + 1$. The assumption we make with regard to the time structure makes no fundamental difference to the analysis so long as we are explicit about it and consistent throughout the model. Therefore, we assume that health-related activities in period t show up in health capital in $t+1$. (If we were working in continuous time, this would not be an issue.) Therefore, our equation of motion for health capital is:

$$H_t = (1 - \delta)H_{t-1} + g(M_{t-1}, v_{t-1}, S_{Pt-1} | H_{t-1}) \qquad (4.2)$$

In Eq. (4.2) the rate of depreciation of health capital from one period to the next is represented by δ, so we can think of δ as reflecting the aging process since it says that, if the individual does nothing to maintain his health, he will gradually lose it. For simplicity at this stage of development of the model, we treat delta as a constant, but it could easily be made a function of age or of H. The second part of the expression includes the health production function $g(M_{t-1}, v_{t-1}, S_{Pt-1} | H_{t-1})$. What Eq. (4.2) shows is that the stock of health capital at the beginning of period $t(H_t)$ depends on the amount of health capital carried over from the previous period, after depreciation $((1 - \delta)H_{t-1} = H_{t-1} - \delta H_{t-1})$, plus the amount of additional health capital the individual was able to build through investments in his health capital. These investments can use a range of inputs, including medical care (M_{t-1}), which refers to formal medical services like physician visits and investment in any health-enhancing goods and services purchased in the market (e.g., visits to the gym); individual withdrawals from the non-monetary services of the community (v_{t-1}), that is, use of their individual social capital; and S_{Pt-1}, use of publicly provided private goods (e.g., meals-on-wheels). The marginal productivity of these inputs in producing future additions to the individual's health capital stock is conditional on his level of health capital in the current period. Specifically, g_X (where $X = M, v, SP$) will approach zero as the individual comes closer to perfect health, since the inputs have less and less ability to generate an increase in the individual's stock of health. "Perfect health" refers to an upper limit to an individual's possible healthfulness, but we do not address the issue of whether perfect health itself can increase over time in this chapter.

Just as we wrote an equation for H that reflects the capital nature of H and the possibility of investing in H, so we can write an equation of motion for individual social capital. We assume that the individual can invest in individual social capital by devoting time, h, to social activities and she they can draw down her stock of social capital according to the term v, which we noted enters the health production function. In other words, it is theoretically possible for the individual to use up all of her accumulated individual social capital.

The equation of motion for individual social capital is:

$$S_{Vt} = (1 - \gamma)S_{vt-1} + \theta(H_{t-1})h_{t-1} - v_{t-1} \tag{4.3}$$

Equation (4.3) says that an individual's stock of social capital in period $t(S_{Vt})$ will decay at a rate, γ, which we assume to be small. Basically, S_V is something an individual has to work on if she wants to draw on it in later periods. In the past, when our societies were more agrarian, farmers came together to rebuild a barn lost to fire (a barn-raising). It is likely that, if one assisted a fellow farmer in his hour of need, that farmer would be ready to return the favor should bad luck strike. That is why we represent the individual's contribution to the community by a time measure h, which is multiplied by $\theta(H_{t-1})$, a function that transforms time into investment effort. $\theta(H_{t-1})$ represents the productivity of the individual's contributions (h) in building his stock of individual social capital. We do this because we are measuring investment effort in terms of time so that investment in individual social capital comes out of the same time constraint as leisure time and work time. We measure h in units of time simply because there is no natural unit for measuring investment in individual social capital directly. We include $\theta(H_{t-1})$ because different individuals can be expected to derive different returns from equal amounts of time devoted to investment in individual social capital. We assume that a healthier individual is more effective than a less healthy one at converting h, which is measured in time units, to units of individual social capital. Therefore, we assume that $\theta'(H_{t-1}) > 0$ so that the productivity with which the individual can build his social capital Sv_i increases with his stock of health. The healthier one is, the easier it is for one to make non-monetary contributions to one's community. We assume that there is a one-period lag between h activities and the consequent increase in individual social capital.

In each period the individual is assumed to have to satisfy a budget constraint of the form:

$$wN_t = p_C C_t + p_M M_t \tag{4.4}$$

where N_t is the total time spent working in period t, and w is the hourly wage rate. The individual can spend his period-t income (wN_t) on consumption goods C that can be acquired at a price p_C or on medical-care goods M at a price p_M. We have simplified the model by assuming that there is no borrowing or lending; we could also elaborate on this framework by allowing income to depend on the individual's stock of health.

In addition to the budget constraint, there is a constraint on time:

$$24 = N_t + L_t + h_t \tag{4.5}$$

The total available time in a given period is assumed to be 24 hours, which can be allocated between time spent at work (N_t), time spent engaged in leisure activities (L_t), and time invested in individual social capital, such as participation in a choir or other community group (h_t). The individual is, in a sense, building an entitlement through h, so if she has been an active member in a group for a long time, then she has an entitlement that has been increasing over time.

We can bring all the pieces of this constrained optimization social capital problem together in the form of a dynamic Lagrangean:

$$
\begin{aligned}
\mathcal{L} = \sum \beta^t U &\left(\frac{wN_t - p_m M_t}{p_c}, H_t, 24 - N_t - h_t \right) \\
&- \beta^{t+1} \lambda_{t+1} [H_{t+1} - [1 - \delta] H_t - g(M_t, v_t, S_{p,t} | H_t)] \\
&- \beta^{t+1} \mu_{t+1} [S_{v,t+1} - [1 - \gamma] S_{v,t} - \Theta(H_t) h_t + v_t] \\
&+ \beta^t \xi_{v,t} v_t + \beta^t \xi_{h,t} h_t
\end{aligned} \tag{4.6}
$$

The first-order condition (FOC) for N_t is:

$$\frac{\partial \mathcal{L}}{\partial N_t} = 0: \quad \frac{U_C}{p_c} = \frac{U_L}{w} \tag{4.7}$$

which is the standard FOC for an income/leisure problem: re-written as in (4.8a), it says that at the consumer's equilibrium the marginal rate of substitution between consumption and leisure equals the ratio of the wage to the price of consumption goods. This value of time condition underlies a number of the other FOCs derived from this model.

$$\frac{U_C}{U_L} = \frac{p_c}{w} \tag{4.8}$$

The FOC for M, medical care (and other commodities or activities which are good for your health), is:

$$\frac{\partial \mathcal{L}}{\partial M_t} = 0: \quad \frac{U_{C,t}}{p_c} = \lambda_{t+1} \beta \frac{g_{M,t}}{p_M} \tag{4.9}$$

The left-hand side of the FOC in (4.9) is the term for the utility from the marginal dollar spent on C, from condition (4.8), while the right-hand side has the Lagrange multiplier from the equation of motion for H, leading one period; the discount factor β; g_M, the marginal product of M_t in the production of H_{t+1}; and the price of a unit of M, p_M. This condition says that at the consumer's equilibrium, the value of the marginal dollar spent on C, equals the utility value of the marginal dollar spent on M, where the utility value of the marginal dollar spent on M involves the marginal productivity of M in producing H and the utility value of a marginal unit of H, represented (as we shall see below) by the Lagrange multiplier. The discount factor β is explicitly present because of the time structure we assumed in the equation of motion for H, by which the effect of an increase in M today does not show up in H until tomorrow. We could rewrite (4.9) as

$$\frac{p_M}{p_c} = \lambda_{t+1} \beta \frac{g_{M,t}}{U_{C,t}} \tag{4.9a}$$

where the left-hand side is the slope of the budget line in the C, M space and the right-hand side is the marginal rate of substitution between C and M, with the marginal utility of C directly shown and the marginal utility of M the product of the remaining terms. Therefore, (4.8a) is also a condition of tangency between a budget line and an indifference curve.

Our interpretation of (4.9a) depends on our interpretation of the Lagrange Multiplier λ_{t+1}. To demonstrate, consider the condition

$$\frac{\partial \mathcal{L}}{\partial H_t}: \quad \lambda_t = U_{H_t} + \beta \lambda_{t+1}[1 - \delta] + \mu_{t+1}\beta\theta_H(H_t)h_t \qquad (4.10)$$

The term involving the Lagrange Multiplier μ is new to our model, but the remainder of this equation is standard to the Grossman model. Ignoring the new term for the moment and looking only at the first two elements of (4.10), we see that λ is defined in terms of its own future value. Leading the expression in (4.10) by one period, again implicitly setting the term involving μ to zero, we can define λ_t in terms of U_{Ht}, U_{Ht+1}, and λ_{t+2}. Leading and substituting again, we see that, in the baseline Grossman case, we have:

$$\lambda_t = U_{H_t} + \beta[1 - \delta]U_{H_{t+1}} + \beta^2[1 - \delta]^2 U_{H_{t+2}} + \beta^2[1 - \delta]^2 U_{H_{t+2}} + \cdots$$
$$(4.11)$$

which tells us that λ_t can be interpreted as the value, in terms of addition to maximized lifetime utility in present value terms, of an additional unit of H acquired in period t. The $[1 - \delta]$ terms are there because one unit of H acquired in period t translates into $[1 - \delta]$ remaining units in period $t + 1$, and so on out. In Eq. (4.10) we have the addition of a term in μ, but the multiplier μ is the Lagrange multiplier on the equation of motion for individual social capital, so it can be interpreted as the addition to the maximized lifetime utility of an additional unit of private social capital, and the remaining terms multiplying μ in (4.10) show the effect of an additional unit of H on the marginal productivity of time spent in amassing individual social capital, h. Therefore, Eq. (4.10) tells us that the shadow price of an additional unit of H now has two components — the lifetime direct addition to utility from an additional unit of health capital and the value of that additional unit of H operating through the individual's capacity to accumulate personal social capital. The greater the productivity of h in producing social capital, and the greater the utility value of that social capital, as represented by μ, the larger that additional element in the valuation of H and the greater the incentive the individual will have to amass H relative to the baseline Grossman model.

Looking at the FOC for h, we have:

$$\frac{\partial \mathcal{L}}{\partial h_t} = 0: \quad U_{L,t} = \beta\mu_{(t+1)\theta(H_t)'} \qquad (4.12)$$

which says that the utility value of an additional hour devoted to the production of individual social capital, h, on the right-hand side of the equation, must equal the utility value of the leisure time that is sacrificed for purposes of investing in individual social capital. We can also derive a FOC for v, consumption of individual social capital, remembering that we have assumed here that v can be measured in natural units rather than time units.

The FOC for v is

$$\frac{\partial \mathcal{L}}{\partial v_t} = 0 : \quad \mu_{t+1} = \lambda_{t+1} g_v(t) \tag{4.13}$$

The right-hand side of Eq. (4.13) is the shadow price of a unit of health capital, multiplied by the marginal productivity of v in generating health capital, while the left-hand side is the shadow price of a unit of private social capital. Remembering that consuming v draws down the individual's private social capital, this condition says that, in the consumer's equilibrium, the utility gained from using up some of her private social capital to produce health capital must equal the cost of the private social capital that has been used up, which is defined in terms of the health capital that the social capital could have been used to produce in the future. We emphasize here that private social capital yields no utility in itself; all of its utility is derived from the possibility of using it to produce health in the future. We can derive an equation of motion for the shadow price of private social capital, from:

$$\frac{\partial \mathcal{L}}{\partial Sv_t} : \quad \mu_t = \beta[1 - \delta]\mu_{t+1} \tag{4.14}$$

This equation for the evolution of the shadow price of the state variable has counterparts in many other dynamic problems.

We have not included an expression for the FOC for Petris-type social capital, S_{Pt} because the individual is not being asked to buy Petris-type social capital but it will be provided to him up to a pre-set limit (which might, of course, depend on his state of health H). Therefore, the individual will consume S_P either up to the constraint of his allocation or up to the point at which the marginal productivity of this item in the production of H falls to zero.

We must also allow for the possibility that h and v can be zero, if in any period the individual is neither adding to nor drawing on his stock of individual social capital, and we must take into account the fact that neither v nor h can be negative. (There is nothing preventing the individual from both adding to and drawing down his stock of individual social capital in any period.) In the Lagrangean above, the

Lagrange Multipliers $\xi_{v,t}$ and $\xi_{h,t}$ represent the non-negativity constraints on v and h: So long as v and h are positive the multipliers will be zero, and the FOCs will be as we have written them above. If either v or h hits the non-negativity barrier, its constraint becomes nonzero and becomes active in the relevant FOC.

In the case of v_t, the FOC will become:

$$\frac{\partial \mathcal{L}}{\partial v_t} = 0: \quad \mu_{t+1} = \lambda_{t+1} g_v(t) + \frac{1}{\beta} \xi_{v,t} \qquad (4.15)$$

The multiplier on the non-negativity constraint for v_t will become positive if, even for very low values of v. Since the marginal productivity of any of the inputs into the health production function $g(\cdot)$ depends on H — in that the closer the individual's actual H is to some level that we term perfect health, the smaller the marginal productivity of any input into $g(\cdot)$ — we expect this condition to arise when the individual is in very good health. Similarly, we expect the non-negativity condition on h_t to come in when the individual is in very poor health, so that $\theta(H_t)$ is zero. Taking those two conditions together, we expect to see individuals add to their stock of individual social capital when they are healthy and draw on it when they are unhealthy. While healthy and unhealthy states can appear at any point in the individual's life, when we are looking at a population at large — in a large panel data set, for example — we expect to see more investment in individual social capital by younger people, with older people tending to draw on the results of their past accumulations.

Thinking about the cases in which the non-negativity constraints on h and v might be binding reminds us that an investment problem, whatever type of capital is being invested in, is inherently a dynamic problem. The FOCs that we derived above are expressed in single-period terms in the sense that the only time subscripts that appear in them are t and $t + 1$. The original Lagrangean expression, however, starts with a summation operator, and the summation covers the entire span of the individual's life. In a dynamic problem, the equations of motion for the state variables are included among the FOCs, just as the static budget constraint, for example, is included among the FOCs in the analysis of a static consumption problem. Decisions about investing in health capital today affect health capital tomorrow and into the future at a rate that depends on δ, the depreciation rate on H. These future values of H in turn affect the first-order conditions for our choice variables at period $t + i$ and ahead.

In a one-state variable dynamic optimization problem, we can bring the instantaneous necessary conditions together with the equations of motion for the state variables through the use of a phase diagram. When we move to more than one-state variable (as we have here, by adding individual social capital as a state variable, along with health capital) the phase diagram technique is generally not open to us. We can, however, make some general comments about the lifetime trajectories that emerge from this problem.

In the base case Grossman model, the typical lifetime trajectory for the stock of health capital for an individual who is born with a high value of H involves a gradual decline in H, with terms like M used to control the rate of decline in H according to the FOC (4.8). That FOC includes the term λ_{t+1}, which represents the value, in terms of maximized lifetime utility, of an additional unit of H received in period $t + 1$. That value, as Eq. (4.4) shows, depends in part on δ, the rate of depreciation of H. Our usual simplifying assumption is that δ is a constant, which leads to the usual result of the baseline Grossman model that investment in health by a person who is initially in very good health starts at low values, increases through part of the life course in order to slow the rate of decline in H relative to the rate at which H would decline if δ were left to operate unchecked, and then, as the payoff period for the investment shortens (i.e., as the end of the lifespan approaches), investment in health declines toward zero. It has been argued that this pattern represents a major flaw in the Grossman model because it does not pick up the empirical fact of increased health expenditures in the later years of life. This problem arises not from a flaw in the logic of the base case Grossman model but in the assumption of the constancy of δ: If we make δ a function of age, say, so that δ increases in later years, then the increased natural rate of decline in H will call forth a countervailing increase in health investment in order to slow the decline of H to the optimal rate (recognizing that the problem remains one with a fixed, finite horizon, i.e., that in the long run we all die). Since private social capital, while potentially important in the individual's lifetime health history, almost certainly has a smaller marginal productivity than do other arguments of the $g(\cdot)$ function, we can hypothesize the lifetime trajectory of this form of capital as an adjunct to the trajectory of health capital, H. In conjunction with our interpretation of the non-negativity conditions on v and h and of the FOCs for v and h, this hypothesis will strengthen our earlier argument that we would expect to see individuals' investment in individual social capital at high levels while they are young and healthy and decrease in later years as the individual's stock of health capital declines. The rate at which H is expected to decline in later years in the absence of individual social capital plays a key role in determining the time patterns of h and v; so long as individual social capital does not naturally depreciate too rapidly through the individual's life, we expect it to be accumulated and stored to be used as a complement to M in the part of the life course closest to the end of the horizon.

This conjecture brings up another issue to which we have given no attention: uncertainty. Strictly speaking, investment problems always involve uncertainty, usually about the payoff to the investment, but the nature of individual social capital adds a twist to this uncertainty. We have treated investment in individual social capital as something the individual does in the same way as he invests in his health capital, but there is a fundamental difference in that the individual's health capital is embodied in the individual himself, whereas social capital is embodied in the community in which the individual lives. Individual social capital is an overlapping-generations concept that takes the form of an individual's having accumulated a record of contributing to his community in the past, usually in the form of providing v services to those who are old when he is young. Investment in individual social capital is, in a sense, an intertemporal version of "do unto others." An individual who has accumulated credit in the community through his actions while young will be able to draw on his accumulated individual social capital in his later years only if the inter-temporal social contract continues to hold, so that younger people, to whom he has not contributed v, will nonetheless contribute v to him as part of the process by which they accumulate their own individual social capital. His v_t is a transformation of their h_t, but they will contribute h only if they expect to be able to draw on other, as yet unborn, individuals' future h when they need to make use of nonzero levels of v. Investment in individual social capital, then, requires that the overlapping generations' social contract holds and is expected to hold in the future, and the return to supplying h will be greater as that social contract is observed more broadly. In some communities the social contract might be observed only within families since families generally have mechanisms by which they can punish individuals who renege on the contract, while in other communities the contract may extend well beyond individual families.

In a reasonably stable and coherent community, an individual's actions in terms of investing in social capital will be reasonably well known. In that type of community, it will be in the interest of younger individuals to contribute h to the community since failure to do so leads, in effect, to ostracism, to their being denied v when they need it. In less stable communities, however, the record-keeping will be more difficult.

By "less stable," we do not necessarily mean dysfunctional. The more geographically mobile a population, the less likely that an individual will stay in one community throughout his entire life, and the less likely he is to be in a position to draw on his investment in individual social capital. Therefore, the expected return from any single individual's investment in his own social capital will be reduced by a factor representing the probability that, by the time he needs to draw on it, he will have moved away. The higher the probability that an individual will not be around to draw on his investment, the less likely he is to invest; in terms of the first-order condition for h, μ will have been reduced significantly, and the immediate return to enjoying leisure will outweigh the expected return to investing in individual social capital, causing the individual to shift his allocation of time away from h and towards L. Since the individual will still plan to follow basically the same lifetime trajectory of health capital, this circumstance tends to lead to greater use of M in the future.

While we noted above that we have not included a FOC for Petris-type social capital since consumption of S_P will be at one of two constraints, either equal to the maximum allocation to which the individual is entitled or equal to the level at which the marginal productivity of Petris goods and services will equal zero — we can say something about the role of Petris social capital in this model. One observation is that S_P and S_V are likely to be closer substitutes for each other than either is for M. Since the individual accumulates S_V while the community provides S_P, the impact of the substitutability is not as straightforward as it would be if the individual were accumulating entitlement to S_P as well as to S_V; but expectations about future access to S_P can be expected to affect the individual's decisions about investing in S_V. We expect that, in communities where more S_P is provided by the community with no significant residency requirement for drawing on S_P, and where that situation is expected to hold in the future, there will be less investment in S_V, which will show up as people's being less involved in community activities (at least those that could be regarded as part of the inter-generational social contract) and more likely to substitute other leisure-time activities for h-type activities. Awareness of reduced investment in S_V because of increased geographic mobility might also lead to communities' deliberately providing more S_P, in which case we expect to observe a dynamic process involving the community's moving over time toward an equilibrium that has less S_V and more S_P, that is, toward more "bowling alone." One implication is that, the more the state does, the weaker the social bonds will be.

Empirical Implications

What the theoretical model makes clear is that we must study social capital at the individual level in a dynamic framework and that we must take account of dynamic interactions among different types of social capital and M-type variables. The model we have proposed here puts social capital into a Grossman investment in health framework, so it must be empirically tested within that framework.

One obvious problem with implementing a forward-looking lifetime intertemporal optimization model is that, relative to the span of an individual's decision horizon, our panel datasets are shortpanel datasets, many of which have observations on large numbers of individuals at many stages in the life course. Absent long panels, we must consider that people of different ages are on different segments of their lifetime trajectories, and we must try to include variables that represent their past behavior in investing in H and in S_V as explanatory variables in equations that explain h and v. Empirically, our data need to allow us to distinguish between h and v using questions not just about feelings of attachment but also about contributions and withdrawals.

Ideally, we want to include variables that affect expectations about the likelihood of earning a return on h, such as social cohesion variables and individual mobility variables. It is also important in a system that analyzes h and v to include S_P-type variables.

Clearly, we are dealing with choices that people make simultaneously, analogous in a sense to the choices firms make about input and output levels. Issues of endogeneity have emerged in the social capital and health literature, and we think that modeling the simultaneous decisions in a dynamic context will help disentangle some of the econometric issues that have been raised.

Socio-economic gradient questions play a major part in the social capital literature. In the context of our model, the wage rate is a key element in determining the opportunity cost of investing in social capital. For example, as female labor force opportunities improved over time, the cost of investing in the social contract increased, which led to a shift away from accumulation of S_V and a greater reliance on M. It is also possible that, for people in lower income segments of the community, the opportunity cost of investing in S_v will be lower, making such investment more attractive and leading to more greater evidence of social cohesion in lower than in higher-income communities. We need to keep in mind, though, that lower-income communities may also have lower values of H, which would lead to a negative relationship between S_V and H at any point across communities at any point in time. This is simply a reminder that we need to consider the accumulation of S_V and H as joint decisions in a lifetime optimization problem. The fact that differences in income level can affect individuals' decisions about investments in individual social capital, which affect health, means that we need to take care in empirical work to disentangle these effects from the effects of the public good type of social capital (e.g., relative income inequality in a community) on health.

A related empirical issue that we have not addressed explicitly in our model is the quality of individual social capital as it relates to the networks to which people belong. Higher-income individuals might either inherit or have easier access to higher-quality social networks, so they may have more productive individual social capital. Just as individuals can be born with high or low values of H, they can be born with high or low values of social capital that are due to the extent of inherited family connections. In our model we have implicitly assumed the initial value of S_V is zero, but it could be much higher, and the lifetime trajectory of investment in social capital would change accordingly.

If the social capital literature is to live up to its potential, we need to devote effort to conceptualizing, refining, and testing empirically specific models of investment in social capital and its impact on health. This chapter suggests that the Grossman framework, which is already a dynamic optimization framework, is a logical starting point for this research program. While there is still much work to be done in specifying the testable hypotheses that come out of the framework we propose, the potential for challenging empirical research based on this framework is promising.

References

Arrow, K. J. 2000. Observations on social capital. In *Social Capital: A Multifaceted Perspective*, eds. Dasgupta P. and Serageldin I., Washington, DC: World Bank: pp. 3–5.
Brown, T. T. and Scheffler, R. M. 2006. The empirical relationship between community social capital and the demand for cigarettes. *Health Economics*, 15(11): 1159–1172.
Folland, S. 2008. An economic model of social capital and health. *Health Economics, Policy and Law*, 3: 333–348.
Grossman, M. 1972. On the concept of health capital and the demand for health. *Journal of Political Economy*, 80(2): 223–255.
Putnam, R. D. 2000. *Bowling Alone: The Collapse and Revival of American Community*, New York: Simon & Schuster.

Solow, R. M. 2000. Notes on social capital and economic performance. In *Social Capital: A Multifaceted Perspective*, eds. Dasgupta P. and Serageldin I., Washington, DC: World Bank: pp. 6–12.

Wilkinson, R. 1996. *Unhealthy Societies: The Afflictions of Inequality*, London: Pyschology Press.

Chapter 5

How Does Social Capital Arise in Populations?

Sherman Folland and Tor Iversen

To enhance the benefits of social activity in populations, one must first understand its sources and their relation to people and culture. Much good work has been done on these topics, and future research will benefit from beginning on the basis of existing theory and evidence. The most salient categories, which form the six parts of this chapter, are age, marital and/or cohabiting status, culture, gender, education, and income. These may also prove the most influential in deriving the production function of social capital. For each category we inquire: "How is this category related to social capital?"

Social Capital and Age

As we age, fewer years remain in which we can enjoy the fruits of our investments. The dynamic investment model developed by Glaeser, Laibson, and Sacerdote (2002) incorporates this fact and predicts that investments in social capital will decline over the lifecycle. Individuals who start out life with low levels of social engagement, the authors reason, may invest heavily at first, but eventually the dynamic changes so as to diminish these investments over time until eventually the depreciation rate exceeds the investments. Thus, theory suggests that social capital will follow an inverted U-shaped pattern over the individual's lifecycle.[4]

Glaeser and colleagues (2002) chose club memberships as their empirical measure of social engagement. Figure 5.1 illustrates this pattern from their empirical data.

---

[4]In an alternative model, the authors derived the conditions for a steady state given an infinite life span. This variation generates different solutions, which may depend on the social capital history of the community and its culture.

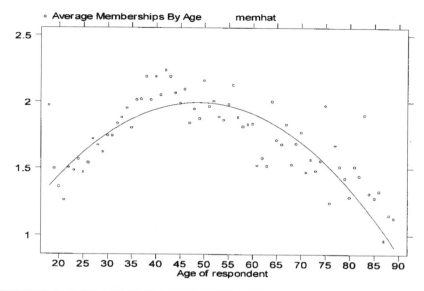

Figure 5.1: Age and Social Capital.
Source: Glaeser, Laibson, and Sacerdote (2002).

The choice of membership as the social capital measure corresponds reasonably well to other social capital research. Putnam (2000) included memberships in his Social Capital Index, and memberships are commonly used elsewhere in research, such as in Brown and colleagues (2006) and Saffer (2008). However, other variables, such as *trust* and the *size* of one's social network tend to perform better in empirical studies of the effects of social capital.

Trust and age

Trust is usually measured by means of surveys that ask the subject to respond to a statement like "I think that other people can usually be trusted." Degree of trust then becomes the score on a Likert scale from strongly Agree = 5 to strongly Disagree = 1. The method does not generate a metric scale, so some see it as less concrete and reliable than metric measures like income and body mass. Trust wins wide acceptance for two reasons: Economists recognize the concept of trust as vital for efficient market exchange (Arrow, 1972), and even this simple measure generates robust results when predicting many health outcomes, especially those related to social and psychological well-being (Niemenin, 2010). Regardless of whether trust holds a central place in a study, it typically appears on social capital studies' lists of variables or in an index (Putnam, 2000).

Trust measures serve well as predictors of an individual's well-being, so it is of interest to determine how a person's trust level changes as he or she ages. Two phenomena are observed from such study: Trust increases from youth to young adulthood and then plateaus, and early cohorts of people exhibit more trusting responses than their replacement cohorts.

Both phenomena are recorded by Robinson and Jackson (2001), who use the General Social Survey for 1972 through 1998 and summarize three groups of trust questions to form their final trust variable. Unlike the data on club memberships over the lifecycle, they find that trust shows no decline late in life, as even those past 80 years of age maintain it. Their more surprising finding is that cohorts decline in trust over the decades. As the authors observe, "Generations born up to the 1940s exhibit high levels of trust, but each generation born after that is less trusting than the one before" (Robinson and Jackson, 2001, p. 117).

This cohort pattern is illustrated in Figure 5.2, which shows the mean trust level for cohorts born in the periods shown along the horizontal axis; sampling periods are indicated on the right. These overlapping cohorts could explain the reported decline

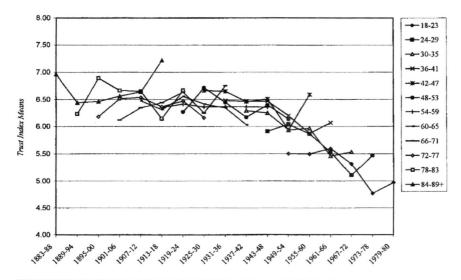

Figure 5.2: Cohort trends in trust in the United States (within age groups).

Source: From Robinson and Jackson (2001).

in social capital in the latter half of the 20th century (Putnam, 2000). Wilkinson and Pickett (2010) also suggest — and support with evidence — the hypothesis that the growth of US income inequality during the last three decades has aggravated the decline in trust. Their data clearly show that trust and income inequality are negatively associated across countries and across the American states. We will return to these associations in the section on income inequality.

Age and trust game experiments

The Investment Game, used in many game theoretic experiments, typically requires the game manager to give n tokens of some value to Player A, who must give some of the tokens to Player B, after which the manager triples A's gift to B. Player B then must return an amount back to A, at which time the play stops. The amounts the players choose to give and give back reflect the degree of trust and reciprocity respectively. Clearly, both players can improve their lot, but if they feel no trust in each other, then the Nash Equilibrium strategy is for A to transfer nothing, and the game is over even as it begins. When older people take the role of Player A, is the result greater or less trusting gifts to B?

The reported results on trust and age for game experiments are generally supportive of the survey results we have described. Sutter and Kocher (2007) study subjects from eight-year-olds to retirees and find that trust increases significantly up to young adulthood, at which point there are no significant differences between further cohorts. Garbarino and Slonim (2009) find similar age patterns for trust, although the cohorts are smaller and cover a tighter set of age cohorts.

Age and social networks

Van Tilburg (1998) reports that the number of friends and relatives people maintain in their social networks remains fairly stable as they age. However, among the Dutch people studied, all of the "old age" subjects shifted gradually toward contacts with their children and away from friends and other relatives; children were the most steadily represented group in a parent's network throughout the part of the lifecycle studied. This pattern can be related to poor health, as children provide informal care to their parents.

Deaton (2009) reports that, for women especially, religious affiliation becomes more important as they age. Religious membership is a form of "social club" that has been shown to have important effects on health and on behaviors risky to health (Brown *et al.*, 2006).

In general, social networks are important to the elderly. Pinquart and Sorenson (2000) conduct a meta-analysis of 286 empirical studies and find that contacts with friends, relatives, and children were significant for the social well-being of the elderly. Overall, however, it is the quality of the relationships that matter, over and above the quantity.

Marriage and Cohabiting[5]: The Demand for Marriage

Marriage can be understood as a social interaction demanded by utility-maximizing individuals. Saffer (2008) derives this type of model, following the original work by Becker (1965) that describes the production of home-produced goods that deliver utility. Let the individual's utility function be

$$U = U(Z_i, Z_j) + \lambda(F - \pi_i Z_i - \pi_j Z_j) \qquad (5.1)$$

where the Z goods are produced by the individual with time and other resources. Let Z_i refer to marriage, and let Z_j refer to some other home-produced good. Let π_I be the full price of marriage and π_j be the price of the other good. "Full price" here refers to all opportunity costs, money costs, and time costs, so it includes the possible lowering of income.

Optimizing on this problem generates a demand function for marriage, Z_i. This demand depends on own price, the price of the other Z good, full income F, and taste:

$$Z_i = Z(\pi_i, \pi_j, F, \text{ and taste}) \qquad (5.2)$$

As Saffer points out, the demand for Z_i is inversely related to its own price; the price of Z_i is a positive function of the wage and the price of purchased goods, and it is a negative function of the marginal product of time and the marginal product of market goods (Saffer, 2008, p. 1050). The author is suggesting that, if one makes

---

[5]We use "marriage" to refer to both traditional marriage and cohabitation in marriage-style partnerships. The theories apply to either type of relationship, although differences are found in comparing some family structures. For examples of these, see Ravenera and Rajulton (2009).

a larger income per hour, the time requirements of marriage may detract from income.

Marriage as a form of social capital

By describing marriage as a "social interaction" that provides gains in utility, we can interpret Z_i as being similar to social capital. This approach is consistent with the seminal writings of Loury (1977) and Coleman (1988), and Putnam (1995, p. 65) states that "the family is the most fundamental unit of social capital." Some may be uncomfortable in describing the marriage relationship as "social," but while its bond is usually stronger and more intimate than other bonds with relatives, friends, and community, it is similar as a bonding relationship. Like other forms of social capital, it benefits health and, in the same way, it provides information, it provides support, and by increasing one's value of life, it encourages life-preserving (risk-avoiding) behaviors.

Isolating marriage effects

These studies suggest overwhelming benefits to marriage, but there are substantial limits to the inferences one can make from them. The principal issue is the difficulty in distinguishing selection (or "sorting") effects from marriage effects.

Prospective marriage partners prefer mates who are relatively healthy and sociable, and who exhibit few bad habits, such as smoking or excessive drinking. Marriage may also bring behavioral improvements, as a study of the anti-social characteristics of young males (Burt, 2011) illustrates. Studying a sample of young men longitudinally, Burt shows that men selected for marriage tend to have fewer anti-social tendencies than those who remain single and that during a few years of marriage the men exhibit further declines in antisocial characteristics. Selection effects and marriage effects made approximately equal contributions to Burt's numerical scale.

The studies of the effects of marriage seldom, if ever, separate the two effects, whether by applying instrumental variable methods or by other means, such as a natural experiment. We cannot assume that our literature's health results for marriage are, like the Burt study, evenly split between the selection effects and the marriage effects, as econometrically, marriage has remained endogenous.

The appearance in the family of children may be less related to selection effects than are marriage effects. A stringent study of the effects of children (Corman *et al.*, 2006) describes the addition of a disabled child as the exogenous family event and the probability of criminal acts by the father before and after the birth of the child. We can understand this event as a disturbance in the social capital of marriage, as the results showed an increase in criminal activity after the birth.

Marriage and other social activity

A strong bonding relationship may turn its members inward so they maintain fewer outside contacts (Bloch, 2007). The evidence on whether this hypothesis applies to marriage is mixed. Groot *et al.* (2007) define a "social network" as "the number of households in your neighborhood [that] you associate with," and they define a "social safety net" as "people you can fall back on." Both the social network and the social safety net are significantly larger for married people, but the result does not hold for club memberships, a result supported by Saffer's (2005) study, where social capital is measured mainly in terms of memberships. In the large majority of groups studied, the marriage indicator associates negatively and significantly with memberships.

Culture and Social Capital

Voluntary cooperation is easier in a community that has inherited a substantial stock of social capital, in the form of norms of reciprocity and networks of civic engagement (Putnam, 1993, p. 167).

The puzzle of Italian civic community

Putnam's study, *Making Democracy Work: Civic Traditions in Modern Italy* (1993), opened a path to understanding quantitatively the importance of civic society to the effectiveness of government institutions. The "civic community" index developed in the study is based on voting patterns, newspaper readership, and the prevalence of sports and assorted associational clubs. The index reveals a striking correlation of civic community with government performance, percentage of voters favoring the republican form of government (as opposed to monarchy), the percentage favoring electoral reform, and the percentage of citizens who are satisfied with government. Putnam identifies the study's findings with the "social capital" developed by Loury (1977), Coleman (1988), and Bordeaux (1985). This work set the stage for Putnam's later research on the United States (2000), which included the health effects of social capital.

Putnam (1993) reveals a distinctive North/South pattern of civic community in regions of Italy, with northern regions obtaining superior outcomes. Putnam hypothesized that the reasons for the differences were historical: Whereas the southern region shined in the years *ca*. 1200AD, its success was built on excellent but autocratic and hierarchical monarchy. In contrast, the cities in the North developed in the 1300s a republican "horizontal" civic community. Could the benefits of this ancient civic boost have lasted more than 500 years to account for Putnam's findings?

A mathematical model and simulation by Guiso, Sapienza, and Zingales (2007) suggests that the answer is "yes." According to the construction of the model, individuals exist in stages of overlapping generations, so parents affect their children's expectations on whether other people can be trusted. As adults, they play a Prisoner's Dilemma game with peers in the community in which they either "defect" (do not cooperate) or "cooperate." As in any Prisoner's Dilemma game, the best joint outcome occurs when both parties cooperate, but there is a built-in tendency to defect, and by experiencing uncooperative opponents, adults will lower their opinions about the trustworthiness of other people. The model, run to simulate many generations of results, finds that "societies can be trapped in a low-trust equilibrium," but a positive shock, such as northern Italy's 14th century republican experience could have had the long-term benefit that Putnam speculates.

"Mapping" Social Capital

The Italy study and its follow-ups were seminal in developing the approach many health economists use today. They also dug deeply into the history and politics of the regions they examine. By "mapping" social capital patterns in both Europe and the United States, we reveal similar puzzles to be explored.

First, there is a strong North/South pattern in social capital in both European countries and across the US states. The European data are illustrated in Table 5.1, and the US data is illustrated in a county-based map of the United States (Figure 5.3).

We label the World Values Survey "trust" variable as trust = 1 if the subject responds positively to the question, "Would you say that most people can be trusted?" and as trust = 0 if the subject responds positively to the statement that with most people you "need to be very careful." To reveal the North/South gradient, we also record the latitude of the capital of each country, which range from 90 degrees

Table 5.1: Average trust in European countries by latitude, World Values Survey.

Country	Average Trust	Latitude	Number of Subjects
Norway	0.742	60.5	1,018
Sweden	0.680	60.1	963
Finland	0.588	61.9	1,001
Switzerland	0.511	46.8	1,187
Netherlands	0.444	52.1	996
Germany	0.341	51.2	1,898
Britain	0.304	55.4	1,022
Italy	0.292	41.9	953
Bulgaria	0.220	42.7	883
Romania	0.203	45.9	1,685
Spain	0.199	40.5	1,184
Poland	0.195	51.9	955
France	0.186	46.2	996
Slovenia	0.181	46.2	999
Serbia	0.153	44.0	1,086
Cyprus	0.128	35.1	1,037
Canada	0.421	56.1	2,107
United States	0.395	37.1	1,241
Mexico	0.155	23.6	1,548

Note: Data on trust and number of subjects were derived from the World Values Survey, 2005. Latitudes are for the capital city of each country.

in the north to 0 degrees at the equator. The correlation coefficient between Average Trust and Latitude is 0.800, indicating a strong North-to-South gradient.

The United States exhibits a similar North/South pattern, seen by examining the county map in Figure 5.3. Social capital density is highest in the north central region, extending out to the Pacific coast and including the northeast.

The causes of these North/South gradients are not well understood. In the United States the gradient may reflect the complex patterns among European immigrations, although this is not likely to be a complete explanation. After all, in that case, what are its original sources of European patterns? New research on population heterogeneity may offer an explanation.

Social Capital and Ethnic Diversity

Several studies find empirical support for greater diversity reducing the level of trust (Dincer, 2010; Leigh, 2006), although trust is also reduced by lower socio-economic status (Letki, 2008).

County-level social capital levels, 1997

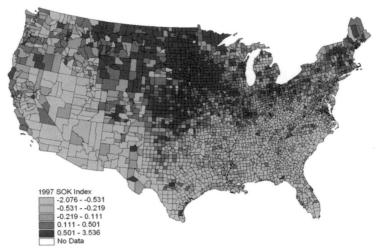

Figure 5.3: Social capital by US County (1997).
Source: Rupasingha, Goetz, and Freshwater (2006).

The issues are thoroughly covered by Putnam (2007). Drawing from the Social Capital Benchmark Survey (2000) of 41 sites in the United States, Putnam derives the result that people in areas with largely homogeneous populations tend to trust other people, even people from other races, more than do those in areas with heterogeneous populations. Figure 5.4 shows Putnam's scattergram results of the pattern of ethnic homogeneity measured by the Herfindahl Index[6] compared to "trust in neighbors" (Putnam, 2007, p. 148).

Putnam (2007, p. 164) concludes that the migration of diverse peoples reduces social capital in the short run, while over longer periods diversity provides a richness in creativity and productivity: "Since the long-run benefits of immigration and diversity are often felt at the national level (scientific creativity, fiscal dividends, and so forth), whereas the short-run costs (frail communities, educational and health

---

[6]The Herfindahl Index is measured on a scale of 0.0 to 1.0, where values are low when there are many small, heterogeneous ethnic groups, and they increase toward 1.0 as a few or one group monopolizes the population.

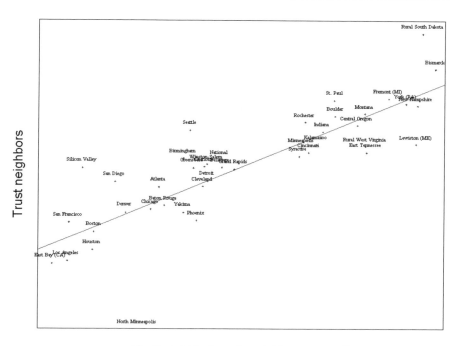

Herfindahl index of racial homogeneity

Figure 5.4: Illustration of the positive correlation between ethnic homogeneity and trust in neighbors.
Source: Putnam (2007, p. 148).

costs) are often concentrated at the local level, there is a strong case for national aid to affected communities."

Education and Social Capital

Some studies show a positive link between education and health, while others find a positive relationship between social capital and health. In this part of the chapter, we study the association between education and social capital since a positive relationship would help to explain the link between education and health.

Education might improve social capital because the knowledge that comes from study and classroom interaction may improve one's understanding of other people, as well as the norms and subcultures in the society. Educated people may be less suspicious and more trusting of other people than less educated people, and more trust makes it easier to join organized community activities.

One might also argue that social capital impacts education, as when parents transfer to children the value and meaning of education or make it easier for their children to obtain information about available types of education. Perhaps social capital also makes it easier to gain admission to the kind of education one prefers. Hence, there might well be an interaction over time, as social capital promotes education, which promotes further accumulation of social capital. There may also be unobserved heterogeneity that impacts both education and social capital, as people who are willing to wait to obtain a reward, such as those who invest in education, may invest in both social capital and human capital.

Many studies examine the relationship between education and social capital. Glaeser *et al.* (1999) present results from regressions across countries using data from the World Values Survey. Consisting of a random sample of 500–3,000 persons in each country covered, the data reveal that education increases both trust and organization membership. Glaeser *et al.* (2002) claim that an individual's decision to accumulate social capital can be analyzed in a standard investment model. They consider social capital as a component of human capital that adds to an individual's market and non-market pay-offs in the future. Like other types of capital, social capital depreciates over time. From the first-order condition of the dynamic maximization problem, the authors find that investment in social capital increases with the occupational returns to social skills. For their empirical work, Glaeser *et al.* (2002) use responses to organization membership questions from the US General Social Survey to find a positive association between the sociability of an occupation and the number of organizational memberships. They also find a uniformly positive relationship between education and social capital investments. However, the interpretation of this association from an investment perspective is not so straightforward, as individuals who do not heavily discount the future are likely to invest in both education and social capital. The existence of a confounding mechanism that is due to time preference makes it less meaningful to state that education leads to social capital from a dynamic perspective.

Saffer (2008) finds the social capital concept unclear and claims that the concept of social interaction is better at capturing the phenomena in which he is interested. Social interaction includes engagement either in organized membership groups or in visiting friends or family. The distinction, since social interaction is described by most of the same variables that describe social capital, is applied to change the theoretical focus compared to previous contributions. Instead of an investment model, as in social capital theory, Saffer treats social interaction as something consumers demand and argues that these engagements once had an important investment motive since both market-based and public insurance were less developed than they are today. Today, social interactions are more of an end in themselves than they once were, because of the pleasure or utility derived from them. Hence, social interactions are consumption goods, and as with other goods, they are produced by market goods and one's own time as inputs, suggesting a kinship with Grossman's theory (1972). The demand for social interaction depends on the price of one's time, the price of other goods, one's taste, and one's full income. These interactions are time-intensive goods, so if education increases the marginal product of one's own time more than it does the marginal product of market goods, education will increase the demand for social interactions. Having tested these predictions empirically with data from the US General Social Surveys (GSS), Saffer finds that education enhances the probability of all memberships and activities except one: visiting activity. Saffer explains the lack of effect on visiting activity as the result of the possible lower effect of education on the marginal product of visiting than that of the other two types of activities. While educated people may become more productive with their time in goal-oriented membership clubs and similar activities, education may not be as relevant for visiting.

A meta-analysis by Huang and colleagues (2009), on the effects of education on social capital assesses data on the results of 65 studies published between 1996 and 2008. In these 65 studies were 154 evaluations on social trust and 286 evaluations on social participation. Huang *et al.* find that one standard deviation in years of schooling accounts for an increase in individual social capital of 12–16 percent in each dimension. They conclude that education is a strong and robust correlate of individual social capital.

Nevertheless, Helliwell and Putnam (2007) express skepticism, noting that in recent US history the education level rose while the stock of social capital reportedly went down and that education is primarily a mechanism for sorting people, as one's participation in clubs may identify one's relative level of education more than it does one's absolute level of education. However, the authors also argue that education has important external benefits in terms of encouraging people to participate more politically and socially when those around them are more educated.

Nie and colleagues (1996) find negative externalities for various types of social engagement and positive effects for social trust, but Helliwell and Putnam (2007) suspect the negative externality result derives from an unfortunate definition of average education that was taken from the national level and argue that the correct definition of average education would be the average level of education in the local community. Helliwell and Putnam (2007) also derive a theoretical argument for a positive externality for participating in clubs or community life: Higher average education helps to create a self-reinforcing climate of trust such that, if individuals know that higher education makes others more trusting, they will likely return the trust to others. Since it is easier to join community life when people are thought to be trustworthy, there is likely to be a positive externality of education on social involvement as well. In order to study the issue empirically, the authors apply a pooled time series and cross-sectional survey data from the United States and find that increases in one's own education and average education both increase trust. They also find for several measures of social engagement that one's own education increases participation, while the average level of education in general has an insignificant effect.

Glaeser *et al.* (2002) state, "The connection between social capital and human capital is one of the most robust empirical regularities in the social capital literature. Better understanding this connection should be a key goal for future research." While their statement still seems to be valid and the association between social capital and human capital is fairly well-established, there is still room for new empirical research on the causal effect of education on social capital.

Gender and Social Capital

Since gender is a true exogenous variable, one may expect that any effects of gender on social capital are causal. However, gender may interact with the environment, so effects of male and female gender on social capital may differ, and these effects may each differ across societies such that it is challenging to distinguish the effect of society from the effect of gender.

Christoforou (2011) studies the formation of social capital across European countries using data from about 100,000 individuals from the European Community Household Panel (ECHP), Wave 6, 1999, which covers a sample of European countries from the former EU-15. The study uses group membership as a dichotomous variable indicating social capital and analyzes associations between explanatory variables and group membership by means of logistic regression. The author finds that being male increases the probability of group membership for the pooled European sample by approximately 40 percent. Coefficients are smallest — showing a decrease in the odds of 10–20 percent — for the Netherlands, Denmark, the UK, and Finland. The results suggest that the impact of being female on group membership depends on the type of society. The marriage coefficient is positive and twice as high for men than for women, suggesting that women often face a tradeoff between family roles and participating in formal social organizations outside the household.

The results of Christoforou (2011) support those of Glaeser *et al.* (2002). Applying data on organizational membership from the General Social Survey in the United States from 1972 to 1998, Glaeser *et al.* (2002) find that social capital incurs a robust negative effect from the indicator for female. The General Social Survey is a repeated annual cross-section of 1,200 to 2,500 respondents.

Bellemare and Kröger (2007) study the effects of trust in a representative sample drawn from the Dutch population. The design closely follows the investment game, in which a potential sender is given an endowment of money and must decide how much to send to the receiver. The experimenter then doubles the amount sent and adds it to the endowment of the receiver. The receiver then decides how much to return to the sender. In addition to these decisions, various background variables are recorded for each participant. The results show that female senders average a higher amount of money than male senders do, but male receivers return a higher amount on average than female receivers do. In general, the higher the amount invested by the sender, the higher the amount returned by the responders. One interpretation of these results is that women send more because they trust that there will be a positive response. On the other hand, women respond less positively than men in the second stage, after which no further response takes place.

Thöni and colleagues (2012) apply experimental methods to the question concerning whether the results from the standard trust question ("Generally speaking, would you say that most people can be trusted or that you can't be too careful in dealing with people?") are good proxies for social capital. They report results from a public-good experiment with randomly selected participants from the Danish population. In the standard one-shot public-good game, participants are endowed with approximately US$10 each and are placed in groups of four people. Each person in each group decides simultaneously how much to give to a common project, at which point all contributions are doubled and shared equally among the four participants. "Don't contribute" is the individually money-maximizing strategy, but if participants trust that the others will contribute, they can substantially increase their money by contributing all of their money. Participants also answer the standard trust questions and share information about individual characteristics. The results show that participants who answer that they trust other people contribute more than people who answer that they do not. Being a female contributes negatively to the amount given when gender is entered as the only control variable, but when it is entered with other control variables, such as age and education, gender is no longer statistically significant. A reasonable conclusion from the study is that we cannot assume that gender has no impact on the willingness to contribute in the simple public-good game.

Croson and Gneezy (2009) review the literature on gender differences in economic experiments, including a number of trust experiments. They find that women trust less than men in some settings but that they trust the same as men in others. They also find that women's trust levels are more context-sensitive than are those of men. In short, women are neither more nor less socially oriented than men, but their social preferences are more situation-specific than are those of men.

The extant empirical studies on gender and social capital show that women have fewer memberships in organizations, as revealed in surveys, while the results of experimental studies about trust are mixed when it comes to the gender component.

Income and Social Capital

The relationships between income, income inequality and social capital tend to be complicated. Societies that feature strong relationships and networks among their people are likely to have a lower degree of income inequality, as people with close connections are likely to prefer income equality. Homogeneous societies with a low level of income inequality may facilitate the formation of social capital in terms of both trust and social activities. The literature contains studies of mechanisms that work in both directions.

Kawachi *et al.* (1997) do a cross-sectional study based on data from 39 US states. Social capital is measured by weighted responses to two items from the General Social Survey: Per-capita density of membership in voluntary groups in each state and level of social trust, measured as the proportion of residents in each state who believe that people can be trusted. The authors find that income inequality is strongly negatively correlated with both per-capita group membership and social trust.

Alesina and La Ferrara (2000) set up a theoretical model to explore the relationship between heterogeneity (including income heterogeneity) and participation in various types of groups. When there is only one homogeneous group, they find that, if a stable equilibrium exists, an increase (decrease) in heterogeneity reduces (increases) total participation. If more than one group exists, the results are more mixed. Testing the theory with data from the US General Social Survey for the years 1974–1994 and estimating models using individual-level data and taking Metropolitan Sampling Areas (MSA) and Primary Metropolitan Sampling Areas (PMSA) as their "community" dimension, the authors find that, after controlling for many individual characteristics, participation in social activities is significantly lower in more unequal and in more racially or ethnically fragmented localities. In Alesina and La Ferrara (2002) the authors show that these results hold when trusting others is used as an indicator of social capital. The amount of personal income adds to the level to which individuals trust others, while income inequality pulls in the opposite direction.

Rupasingha *et al.* (2006) follow up on Alesina and La Ferrara (2000) with data at the level of US counties. They use an array of individual and community variables they consider to be theoretically important determinants of social capital and find that homogeneity in general is positively associated with levels of social capital across US counties. However, they do not find a statistically significant effect of income inequality.

Fischer and Torgler (2006, 2007) study whether an individual's relative income position has an effect on his or her stock of social capital. They distinguish the multiple facets of social capital along four dimensions: Trust between people, the people's confidence in institutions, compliance with social norms, and the creation of networks. They hypothesize that a disadvantageous relative income position is detrimental to an individual's trust in societal institutions like the courts, Parliament, business, and industry and that it is deleterious to individuals' willingness to obey the law, comply with norms, and participate in voluntary activities. The empirical analysis makes use of individual cross-section data from the 1998 ISSP survey, which covers approximately 24,000 observations from 26 countries and provides precise information on personal income. The authors take the possibility of an asymmetric income effect into account by differentiating between the impact for "poorer" persons from that for "richer" persons. The authors admit the possible endogeneity problem in their empirical analysis, saying that because of the cross-sectional nature of the data, reversed causality and measurement error might bias the estimated coefficients. In general, they find empirical support for the relevance of relative income position for social capital. In most cases, they observe that the coefficients that measure a respondent's relative income position are statistically significant, with considerable marginal effects. For the generalized trust measure, social capital rises with relative income.

Groot *et al.* (2007) calculate the compensating income variation of social capital. Data for their empirical analysis are taken from the GPD-survey 2002, done in the Netherlands. They define social capital by the size of the social network and membership in unions or associations and analyze what determines these aspects of social capital. They then calculate the additional income that is required to compensate for the positive effect of social capital on people's well-being and find that the compensating income is substantial.

The literature also contains studies of the effect of social capital on income inequality. Robison and Siles (1999) and Robison *et al.* (2011) study the effect of social capital on household income distribution in US counties in the census years 1980, 1990, and 2000. They define social capital as "a person's or group's sympathy or sense of obligation for another person or group." Their model implies that increased social capital increases concern for other people's income and a more equal income distribution in the community. At the empirical level they use a broader set of indicators for social capital than many other studies do; they include measures of family integrity, educational achievement, litigation, and labor force participation. Family integrity is proxied by the percentage of households headed by a single female with children, which the authors argue is a strong indicator of social capital since, all else being equal, the children have access to the social capital associated with each parent. Possible endogeneities, such as that single parents have average lower incomes than two-parent families do, are accounted for by taking the values of lagged explanatory variables. The authors find that an increase in their indicators of social capital increases the mean household income and reduces the variation in household income at the county level. The result that people are more likely to express preferences for income redistribution in areas with higher rates of community participation than in those with lower rates of community participation is supported by a study from Japan by Yamamura (2012).

Taking the published literature together, it is reasonable to conclude that income inequality prevents a high level of social capital, while social capital promotes less income inequality. Possible self-enforcing effects remain to be studied.

Summary and Concluding Remarks

This book addresses the issue of social capital and health, and several of its chapters argue that social capital is likely to have a positive impact on health. From a policy perspective, then, it is important to understand the factors that contribute to social capital. A chapter about how social capital arises in populations is an important element in how overall health may be improved by promoting the creation of social capital.

This chapter covers a review and discussion of six elements from the literature: age, marriage and cohabitating, culture, education, gender, and income. While the chapter benefits from a literature search in several databases, it does not provide a systematic literature review.

The relationship between age and social capital is generally predicted to follow an inverted u-shape. The downward part of the prediction is related to a declining number of years left to harvest the benefits of social capital and to the increasing cost of investing in social capital as one grows old and frail. The prediction is supported by some empirical studies that use the number of memberships in organizations as the indicator of social capital. On the other hand, trust as an indicator of social capital shows no decline with age.

Marriage and cohabitation can, in itself, be considered a type of social capital. Marriage may also turn to a strong bonding relationship that involves fewer outside contacts, reducing social capital. The empirical literature shows mixed results.

Empirical studies show a North/South pattern in social capital, both across European countries and across US states, and the section about culture and social capital offers some explanations from the literature. We also refer to simulation studies of overlapping generations that suggest that societies can be trapped in a low-trust equilibrium and that both positive and negative shocks may have long-term effects on social capital.

Education may improve social capital for several reasons. Study and classroom interaction may increase one's understanding of other people, as well as the norms and culture in society, so educated people may be less suspicious than uneducated people are and more trusting of other people. Trust also makes it easier to join organized community activities. These predictions are supported by empirical studies; the connection between human capital and social capital is considered to be one of the most robust empirical regularities in the social capital literature.

The results from literature on the relationship between gender and social capital are mixed, but they show an important interaction between gender and society. Women seem to have fewer memberships in organizations than men, while the results from the experimental studies about trust are mixed.

The relationship between income, income inequality and social capital is complex. Homogenous societies with low levels of income inequality may facilitate the formation of social capital in terms of trust and in terms of social networks. A high level of social capital may also lead to a preference for income equality. Taken together, the literature reviewed here suggests that excessive income inequality prevents a high level of social capital in a society.

This chapter reviewed the theoretical and empirical literature concerning the factors that contribute to the creation of social capital. The relationships between these factors and social capital are likely to be complex and often not sufficiently understood as a background for policy interventions. For instance, we argue that education is likely to promote the formation of social capital, but it can also be argued that social capital makes it easier to obtain information and access to appropriate education by means of one's network. The empirical literature has so far concentrated on relationships, rather than on revealing causal effects.

References

Alesina, A. and La Ferrara, E. 2000. Participation in heterogeneous communities. *Quarterly Journal of Economics,* 115: 847–904.

Alesina, A. and La Ferrara, E. 2002. Who trusts others? *Journal of Public Economics*, 85: 207–234.

Arrow, K. 1972. Gifts and exchanges. *Philosophy and Public Affairs*, 1: 343–362.

Becker, G. 1965. Theory of the allocation of time. *Economic Journal*, 75: 493–507.

Bellemare, C. and Kröger, S. 2007. On representative social capital. *European Economic Review*, 51, 183–202.

Bloch, F., Genicot, G. and Ray, D. 2009. Reciprocity in groups and limits to social capital. American Economic Review, Papers and Proceedings, May issue.

Bordieu, P. 1986. The forms in capital. In *Handbook of Theory and Research for the Sociology Education.* New York: Greenwood, pp. 241–258.

Bradford, D. 2003. Pregnancy and the demand for cigarettes. *American Economic Review*, 93(5): 1752–1763.

Brown, T. *et al.* 2006. The empirical relationship between community social capital and the demand for cigarettes. *Health Economics*, 15: 1159–1172.

Burt, S.A. 2011. Does marriage inhibit antisocial behavior? An examination of selection vs causation via a longitudinal twin design. *Archives of General Psychiatry*, 67: 1309–1315.

Christoforou, A. 2011. Social capital across European countries: Individual and aggregate determinants of group membership. *American Journal of Economics and Sociology*, 70: 699–728.

Coleman, J. 1988. Social capital in the creation of human capital. *American Journal of Sociology*, (Supplement) 94: S95–S120.

Corman, H. *et al.* 2006. Crime and circumstance: The effects of infant health shocks on fathers' criminal activity. National Bureau of Economic Research, Working Paper No. 12754.

Croson, R. and Gneezy, U. 2009. Gender differences in preferences. *Journal of Economic Literature,* 47: 448–474.

Deaton., A. 2009. Aging, religion, and health Mimeo, Princeton University. Available at: www.Princeton.edu/-Deaton/downloads/Religion_and_health_all_August09.pdf.

Dincer, O. 2011. Ethnic diversity and trust. *Contemporary Economic Policy*, 29: 284–293.

Fischer, J. A. V. and Torgler, B. 2006. The effect of relative income position on social capital. *Economics Bulletin*, 26: 1–20.

Fischer, J. A. V. and Torgler, B. 2007. Social capital and relative income concerns: Evidence from 26 countries. Berkeley Program in Law and Economics, Working Paper Series, UC Berkeley.

Garbarino, E. and Slonim, R. 2009. The robustness of trust and reciprocity across a heterogeneous population. *Journal of Economic Behavior & Organization*, 69: 226–240.

Glaeser, E., Laibson, D. and Sacerdote, B. 2002. An economic approach to social capital. *The Economic Journal*, 111: 507–548.

Glaeser, E. L., Laibson, D., Scheinkman, J. A. and Scoutter, C. L. 1999. What is social capital? The determinants of trust and trustworthiness. NBER Working Paper 7216. Available at: http://www.nber.org/papers/w7216.pdf.

Groot, W., Maassen van den Brink, H. and van Praag, B. 2007. The compensating income variation of social capital. *Social Indicators Research*, 82, 189–207.

Grossman, M. 1972. On the concept of health capital and the demand for health. *Journal of Political Economy*, 80(2): 223–255.

Guiso, L., Sapienza, P. and Zingales, L. (2008). Long term persistence. National Bureau of Economic Research.

Helliwell, J. F. and Putnam, R. D. 2007. Education and social capital. *Eastern Economic Journal*, 33, 1–19.

Huang, J. 2010. Education and social capital: Empirical evidence from microeconomic analyses. Tinbergen Institute Research Series Book No. 472. Tinbergen Institute, University of Amsterdam, Amsterdam.

Huang, J., Maassen van den Brinka, H. and Groot, W. 2009. A meta-analysis of the effect of education on social capital. *Economics of Education Review*, 28: 454–464.

Kawachi, I., Kennedy, B. P., Lochner, K. and Prothrow-Stith, D. 1997. Social capital, income inequality, and mortality. *American Journal of Public Health*, 87: 1491–1499.

Leigh, A. 2006. Trust, inequality and ethnic heterogeneity. *The Economic Record*, 82: 268–280.

Letki, N. 2008. Does diversity erode social cohesion? Social capital and race in British neighborhoods. *Political Studies*, 56: 99–126.

Nie, N. H., Junn, J. and Stehlik-Barry, K. 1996. *Education and Democratic Citizenship in America*. Chicago, IL: University of Chicago Press.

Nieminen T, *et al.* 2010. Social capital as a determinant of self-rated health and psychological well-being. *International Journal of Public Health*, 55(6): 531–542.

Pinquart, M. and Sörensen, S. 2000. Influences of socioeconomic status, social network, and competence on subjective well-being in later life: A meta-analysis. *Psychology and Aging*, 115(2): 187–224.

Putnam, R. D. 1993. *Making Democracy Work: Civic Traditions in Modern Italy*, Princeton, NJ: Princeton University Press.

Putnam, R. D. 2000. *Bowling Alone: The Collapse and Revival of American Community*, New York: Simon & Schuster.

Putnam, R. D. 2007. *E pluribus unum:* Diversity and community in the twenty-first century: The 2006 Johan Skytte Prize. *Scandinavian Political Studies*, 30(2): 137–174.

Ravanera, Z. R. and Rajulton, F. 2009. Measuring social capital and its differentials by family structure. *Social Indicators Research*, 95: 63–89.

Robison, L. J. and Siles, M. E. 1999. Social capital and household income distributions in the United States: 1980, 1990. *The Journal of Socio-Economics*, 28: 43–93.

Robison, L. J., Siles, M. E. and Jin, S. 2011. Social capital and the distribution of household income in the United States: 1980, 1990, and 2000. *The Journal of Socio-Economics*, 40: 538– 547.

Robinson, R. V. and Jackson, E. F. 2001. Is trust in others declining in America? An age-period-cohort analysis. *Social Science Research*, 30: 117–145.

Rupasingha, A., Goetz, S. J. and Freshwater, D. 2006. The production of social capital in US counties. *The Journal of Socio-Economics*, 35: 83–101.

Saffer, H. 2008. The demand for social interaction. *The Journal of Socio-Economics*, 37: 1047–1060.

Sutter, M. and Kocher, M. G. 2007. Trust and trustworthiness across different age groups. *Games and Economic Behavior*, 59: 364–382.

Thöni, C., Tyran, J.-R. and Wengström, E. 2012. Microfoundations of social capital. *Journal of Public Economics*, 96: 635–643.

Van Tilburg, T. G. 1998. Losing and gaining in old age: Changes in personal network size and social support in a four-year longitudinal study. *Journal of Gerontology: Social Sciences*, 53B: S313–S323.

Wilkinson, R. and Pickett, K. 2010. *The Spirit Level*, London: Penguin.

Yamamura, E. 2012. Social capital, household income, and preferences for income redistribution. *European Journal of Political Economy*, 28: 498–511.

Chapter 6

Measures of Social Capital

Richard M. Scheffler and Yumna Bahgat

We first explore the historical development of social capital and how the conceptualization and the proposed definitions of social capital have evolved over time and continue to develop. Although many scholars and academics have explored the term *social capital*, there are four definitions, as proposed by Bourdieu (1986), Coleman (1988), Putnam (1993, 2000), and the World Bank that have been dominant in the academic debate. The social capital definitions included in the papers of several economists are also explored. The varying definitions and descriptions of social capital point to the fact that there is no one distinct definition, but rather, social capital can be attributed to conceptual and empirical ideas based on social interactions, relations, structures, and values. The empirical measurements of social capital throughout the book are then evaluated in terms of their usefulness in explaining the relationship between social capital and health, based on three criteria.

The application of social capital can also be seen in the health and medical arena, where the number of publications on social capital and its relationship to health, medical care, and mortality has been increasing. This upward trend is analyzed using three literature indices.

Finally, using data from the World Values Survey Questionnaire 2005–2006, we explore the correlation between health and happiness, as well as social capital measures like trust, friendship, and membership in organizations. From these correlations and overall observations on the development of social capital, this chapter seeks to address the future of social capital and health.

What are the Definitions of Social Capital?

The concept of social capital has evolved over time. Many scholars, including those in the fields of sociology, political science, economics, and anthropology, have shaped the historical development of the definition of social capital. In 1920, Hanifan described social capital as something that "makes those tangible substances count for most in the daily lives of people: Namely good will, fellowship, sympathy, and social intercourse among the individuals and families" (Borgatti, 1999). Throughout the years social capital has been further explored and described using a range of terms and phrases, including "networks" (Jacobs, 1961), "friends and acquaintances" (Hannerz, 1969), the "collectivity that affects the economic goals of its members" (Portes and Sensenbrenner, 1993), and the "affiliations … [in] an individual's personal network" (Belliveau, O'Reilly, and Wade, 1996). In the late 20th century, social capital was further defined as the "norms and values that permit cooperative behavior" (Fukuyama, 1997), "the process and conditions among people" (Kreuter, 1998), "the standing one has in a social organization and the concurrent ability to draw on that standing to influence the actions of others" (Friedman and Krackhardt, 1997), "the connectedness with potential clients" (Pennings, Lee, and van Witteloostujin, 1998), "the social trust, norms and networks" (Sirianni and Friedland, 1997), and a concept "rooted in social networks and social relations … as resources embedded in a social structure which are accessed and/or mobilized in purposive actions" (Lin, 1999). The development of social capital definitions carried on into the 21st century, when the Petris Social Capital Index was formed and researchers from UC Berkeley's Nicholas C. Petris Center for Health Care Markets and Consumer Welfare defined social capital through a supply-side measurement of participation in membership organizations (Brown *et al.*, 2008).

A common theme of these definitions, which span several academic disciplines, is that the resources available to individuals and communities are attributed to behaviors and membership in community networks. These descriptions and definitions of social capital throughout history make clear that there is no one concrete definition for the concept. Rather, social capital can be attributed to both conceptual and empirical ideas based on social interactions, relationships, structures, and values.

The Four Basic Definitions of Social Capital

While the term *social capital* has been explored and analyzed by many scholars, four basic definitions that are dominant in the academic debate are frequently applied in various areas of research. Bourdieu (1986), Coleman (1988), and Putnam

(1993, 2000) made significant contributions to the renewed interest in social capital starting in the late 20th century, while the World Bank's definition of social capital is used in their Social Capital Initiative, which explores the development and impact of social capital on the global scale.

In his work titled *The Forms of Capital* (1986), Pierre Bourdieu was one of the first scholars to examine social capital's role sociologically. In his analysis, Bourdieu employed economic and cultural contexts to draw his conclusions. Bourdieu defined social capital as "the aggregate of the actual or potential resources which are linked to possessions of a durable network of more or less institutionalized relationships of mutual acquaintance and recognition — or in other words to membership of a group — which provides each of its members with the backing of the collectivity-owned capital, a credential which entitles them to credit, in the various senses of the word" (Bourdieu, 1986, p. 248). Using a more theoretical approach, Bourdieu connects these ideas on social capital with ideas on class and social inequality, describing how an individual's ability to mobilize networks and social relationships determines the amount of his or her social capital. This interpretation also sheds light on how social capital can be used to preserve and reinforce societal class structures.

In *Social Capital in the Creation of Human Capital* (1988), Coleman focused on the mechanisms and role of social capital in societal structures, incorporating both the social perspective and the economic perspective to navigate the meaning of what it means to have social capital. Coleman stated, "Social capital is defined by its function. It is not a single entity, but a variety of different entities, having two characteristics in common: They all consist of some aspect of a social structure, and they facilitate certain actions of individuals who are within the structure" (Coleman, 1990, p. 302). Coleman's analysis of social capital argues that groups that hold a certain level of trust and trustworthiness can accomplish significantly more than those who do not hold such trust. Coleman's work represents a shift in thinking from Bourdieu's ideas on individual-based outcomes to a more society-based approach that focuses on groups, organizations, and institutions.

Making Democracy Work: Traditions in Modern Italy written in 1993, was another major contributor to the renewed interest in social capital. In this work, which uses a political science lens to explore the effect of reforms in Italy during the 1970s, Putnam found that democracy worked better when there were higher levels of civic engagement and defined social capital as "features of social organizations, such as trust, norms, and networks that can improve the efficiency of society by facilitating coordinated actions (Putnam, 1993, p. 167). Putnam's *Bowling Alone: The Collapse and Revival of American Community* written in 2000, applied the author's social capital analysis to the United States and concluded that schools, neighborhoods, the economy, democracy, health, and happiness depend on adequate amounts of social capital. In defining social capital, Putnam wrote, "While physical capital refers to physical objects and human capital refers to properties of individuals, social capital refers to connections among individuals — social networks and the norms of reciprocity and trustworthiness that arise from them" (Putnam, 2000, pp. 18–19). Putnam used an empirical approach to develop an instrument for measuring an index of civic engagement that is marked by trust in people and institutions, norms of reciprocity, networks, and membership in voluntary associations, which he used to describe social capital in the United States (Figure 6.1). Putnam also distinguished between two types of social capital, bridging and bonding, describing bridging social capital as relationships between groups that bridge diverse social spheres, and bonding social capital as the inward relationships within homogenous groups.

Although Bourdieu, Coleman, and Putnam share similarities in their quests to define and understand social capital, there are also differences in their definitions.

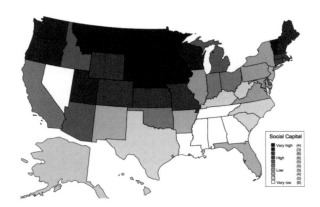

Figure 6.1: Social capital in the American states.

Note: This index is used as a way to measure social capital based on membership in a range of organizations, which reflect an individual's desire for social engagement. The index uses 14 variables, including community or organizational life, engagement in public affairs, volunteerism, and social trust.

Source: Putnam index (Putnam, 2001).

Putnam's definition of social capital emphasizes the collective nature of the concept and its application to the individual level, as well as to the societal and political levels. Bourdieu, on the other hand, emphasized the individual and stressed the different degrees to which individuals have access to networks and how that access translates into the unequal distribution of capital and power. For his part, Coleman viewed organizations and corporations as individuals and stressed that social capital can make up for the lack of human or cultural capital. However, all three of these scholars agreed that one of the main components of social capital is that it encompasses social networks and can lead to beneficial outcomes.

The fourth definition of social capital, which has been influential in analyzing development outcomes, is the World Bank's definition of social capital. According to the World Bank, "Social capital refers to the institutions, relationships, and norms that shape the quality and quantity of a society's social interactions.... Social capital is not just the sum of the institutions which underpin a society; it is the glue that holds them together" (World Bank, 2011). The World Bank, a development agency, seeks to create a supportive environment for the emergence of the social capital that will hold societies together and contribute to economic growth and human well-being.

Social Capital Definitions Used by Economists

In the 2012 Workshop of the Global Network on Social Capital and Health at the University of Padova (Italy), several economists presented papers on the topics of social capital and health that included the following definitions of social capital:

- Berchet, Laporte, and Jusot reported that a key limitation that has been largely recognized by the literature is the lack of clarity about the concept, as "social capital means different things to different people" (Grootaert and Serageldin, 2000). Social capital has been defined by some as a collective resource, and as referring to "features of social organization, such as trust, norms and networks that can improve the efficiency of society by facilitating coordinated actions" (Putnam, 1993). For others, social capital is an individual resource that enables private returns, thanks to interaction with others (Glaeser, Laibson and Sacerdote, 2002).
- Gagliardi, Rosa and Lattanzio (2012) referred to Coleman (1990) and Bourdieu (1986) in adopting in their study "the sociological perspective which

traditionally identifies social capital as an individual resource including social network, support, and trust in local environment and social participation."

- Berchet and Sirven explained that, "Although most of the empirical literature on the determinants of social capital stresses the important role of the economic, political, and social context, only few institutional measures have been used to explain migrants' investment in social capital.... Among the institutional determinants of social capital unexplored for the migrant population, some light should be shed on three main areas: social heterogeneity, non-egalitarian or corrupt societies, and welfare states regimes."

- Corman, Noonan, and Reichman defined social capital as "an individual attribute arising from social networks and relationships rather than as a collective response that is located in the context of a country, region or state. An individual invests in social capital by forming and maintaining social interactions, wherein the returns from this investment yield utility and improve resource allocations (e.g., through information sharing and efficiencies in decision making)."

- Blanchad, Singh and Mignone (2012) explained that the construct of social capital in their study "follows Bourdieu (1992) and Portes (1998, 2000) in theorization and Szreter and Woolcock (2004) and Mignone (2004) in operationalization.... Bonding, Bridging and Linking social capital have been recognized as the three dimensions of social capital.... Following Portes, social capital will mostly have functional role but can have negative effect also. Following Bourdieu, migrants can have differential levels of social capital, depending on the 'actual or potential resources' they possess or can access in the time of need."

- Folland, Islam and Kaarbøe (2012) observed, "Social capital as understood by Loury (1977), Coleman (1990), and Putnam (1993, 1995 and 2000) is a concept of community, friends and family that could achieve social benefits beyond of the paradigm of the neoclassical market and the invisible hand. Health improvement was one of the benefits suggested by Putnam's data, and, since then, research from many disciplines, especially epidemiology, sociology, political science, and more recently health economics, has confirmed this result."

- Fiorillo and Sabatini explained, "Structural social capital deals with individuals' behaviors and mainly takes the form of networks and associations which can be observed and measured through surveys. Cognitive social capital derives from individuals' perceptions resulting in norms, values and beliefs that contribute to cooperation. These latter aspects involve subjective evaluations of the social environment. Both structural and cognitive dimensions include several sub-dimensions whose relationship with health variables in turn varies depending on the context and on the effect of other individual and local potentially influential factors (Moore, Gauvin and Dubè, 2009; Yamamura, 2011)."

- Averette's contribution was that, "Though most view social capital as social organization in the form of trust, norms and values that facilitate economic and social efficiency, the details are much more elusive since social capital is inherently multidimensional."
- Rocco and d'Hombres contributed the view that, "First, social capital, by favoring more intense and frequent social interactions, may support the creation of information channels and help spreading ideas about the harms of tobacco, public health campaign messages, or strategies of smoking cessation. Second, social capital can enhance trust in public and governmental institutions, which are normally in charge of delivering antismoking campaigns."
- Finally, Halla and Zweimuller defined social capital as "social Gradient in the short-term and long-term effects."

Empirical Measures of Social Capital Throughout the Book

We evaluate in general terms the usefulness of measures of social capital in explaining the relationship between social capital and health using three criteria:

1. How the measure related to the theoretical relationship between social capital and health through information and the bridging and bonding through people.
2. How well the measure empirically correlates with various measures of health, both physical and mental.
3. How the measure relates to the conceptual measure of social capital and behaviors. The social capital scores of the various measures found in the chapters of this book range from 1 through 5, with 1 the highest score and 5 the lowest score (Table 6.1).

Upward trend of publications on social capital and health

Social capital research continues to grow and develop, with a significant upward trend currently in the number of papers published that analyze, conceptualize, measure, and apply the theory of social capital in a health and health outcomes context. This explosion of publications regarding social capital and health can be

Table 6.1: Empririical measures of social capital throughout the book.

Chapter	Name of Measure	Concept	Measure	Rating
Chapter 3: "How Do We Invest in Social Capital?" by Folland, Kaarboe, and Islam	Utility Maximization Model of Social Capital and Health	Based on the idea that the choice of social capital interaction entails opportunity costs, primarily in time and lost wages. This measure takes into account the conventional labor/leisure tradeoff.	Utility $= U(S, E, C)$ E = a public good or investment S = enabler of social capital C = other goods Social capital is an endogenous choice variable; to observe the changes in social capital an exogenous public investment is introduced. The chapter also explores the effect of subsidizing the price of higher education.	3
Chapter 4: "Social Capital: An Economic Perspective," by Laporte	Grossman Model	The Grossman framework looks at individuals' health-related decisions from a lifetime perspective and yields predictions about trajectories of health and health-related behaviors through the entire lifespan. The Grossman model is a framework used to incorporate decisions about investment in individual social capital in as much as social capital may affect health.	$S_{Vt} = (1 - \gamma)S_{vt-1}$ $+ \theta(H_{t-1})h_{t-1} - v_{t-1}$ An individual's stock of social capital in period t (S_{Vt}) will decay at a rate γ, which we assume to be small. S_V is something an individual has to work on if he or she wants to draw on it in later periods.	2
Chapter 5: "How Does Social Capital Arise in Populations?" by Folland and Iverson	Social Capital and Age: Dynamic Investment Model	The dynamic investment model developed by Glaeser, Laibson, and Sacerdote (2002) predicts that investments in social capital will decline over the life cycle. The chapter suggests that social capital will follow an inverted U-shaped pattern over a person's life cycle.	Glaeser and colleagues chose club memberships as their empirical measure of social engagement.	1

(Continued)

Table 6.1: (Continued)

Chapter	Name of Measure	Concept	Measure	Rating
	Social Capital and Age: Social Networks	In general, social networks are important to the elderly. Pinquart and Sorenson (2000) conducted a meta-analysis of 286 empirical studies and found that contacts with friends, relatives, and children were significant for the social well-being of the elderly.	The number of friends and relatives one maintains in one's network.	1
	Social Capital and Age: Trust	Trust wins wide acceptance for two reasons: Economists recognize the concept of trust as vital for efficient market exchange (Arrow, 1972), and even this simple measure generates robust results when predicting many health outcomes, especially those related to social and psychological well-being (Niemenin, 2010). Whether trust holds a central place in a study or not, it typically appears as one of social capital's list of variables or in an index (Putnam, 2000).	Trust is usually measured by surveys that ask the subject to respond to a statement of the type, "I think that other people can usually be trusted." Degree of trust then becomes the score on a Likert scale from strongly agree = 5 to strongly disagree = 1.	3
	Marriage	Marriage can be understood as a social interaction demanded by utility-maximizing individuals. Like other forms of social capital, it benefits health and in the same way: it provides information, it provides support, and by increasing one's value of life, it encourages life-preserving (risk-avoiding) behaviors.	$U = U(Z_i, Z_j) + \lambda(F - \pi_i Z_i, -\pi_j Z_j)$ $Z = $ goods are produced by the Individual with time and other resources. $Z_i = $ marriage, $Z_j = $ some other home-produced good. $\pi_I = $ the full price of marriage and $\pi_j = $ the price of the other good. By describing marriage as a social interaction that provides gains in utility, we can interpret the Z_i as being of a kind with social capital.	4

(Continued)

Table 6.1: (Continued)

Chapter	Name of Measure	Concept	Measure	Rating
	Culture: Civic Community Index	Putnam's study, *Making Democracy Work: Civic Traditions in Modern Italy* (1993), opened a path to understanding quantitatively the importance of civic society to the effectiveness of government institutions.	The "civic community" index that Putnam developed is based on voting patterns, newspaper readership, and prevalence of sports and associational clubs.	2
	Ethnic Diversity and the Herfindahl Index	Putnam concluded that the migration of diverse peoples reduces social capital in the short run, while over longer periods diversity increases creativity and productivity.	Drawing from the 2000 Social Capital Benchmark Survey's survey of 41 sites in the United States, Putnam derives the result that people in US cities and areas with more homogeneous populations tend to hold other people, even people from other races, in greater trust than do people from areas with less homogeneous populations. The scattergram results show the pattern of ethnic homogeneity measured by the Herfindahl Index compared to "trust in neighbors" (Putnam, 2007, p. 148). The Herfindahl Index is measured on a scale of 0.0 to 1.0, where low values occur if there are many small ethnic groups and increase toward 1.0 as one or a few groups monopolize the population.	2

(Continued)

Chapter	Name of Measure	Concept	Measure	Rating
	Education	Studies show a positive link between education and health. Many find a positive relationship between social capital and health.	The empirical work uses responses to organization membership questions from the US General Social Survey. The study finds that there is a positive association between the sociability of an occupation and the number of organizational memberships. There is a uniformly positive relationship between education and investments in social capital.	3
	Gender	Gender may interact with the environment, so effects of gender on social capital differ between male and female, and these effects may each differ across societies.	Christoforou (2011) studies the formation of social capital across European countries using group membership as the indicator of social capital. Applying data on organizational membership from the General Social Survey in the United States from 1972 to 1998, the study finds that social capital incurs a robust negative effect from the indicator for female.	3
	Income	Societies with strong relationships and networks between people are likely to have a lower degree of income inequality. People with close connections are likely to prefer income equality. Homogeneous societies with a low level of income inequality may facilitate the formation of social capital in terms of both trust and social activities.	Kawachi et al. (1997) do a cross-sectional study based on data from 39 US states. Social capital is measured by weighted responses to two items from the General Social Survey: Per-capita density of membership in voluntary groups in	

(Continued)

Table 6.1: (Continued)

Chapter	Name of Measure	Concept	Measure	Rating
			each state and level of social trust, measured as the proportion of residents in each state who believe that people can be trusted. The study finds that income inequality is strongly negatively correlated with both per-capita group membership and social trust.	3
Chapter 6: "Measures of Social Capital," by Scheffler and Bahgat	The Petris Social Capital Index (PSCI)	Created by researchers at UC Berkeley's Nicholas C. Petris Center for Health Care Markets and Consumer Welfare, the PSCI provides a supply-side measure of participation in membership organizations.	The index looks at 18 community voluntary organizations using public data available for the entire United States. Investment in these organizations is strongly correlated with physical capital if there is something tangible (church, YMCA) that can be invested in.	1
Chapter 7: "The Empirics of Social Capital and Health," by Rocco and Fumagalli	Health Reduced-form Model	Grounded on Grossman's model, the empirical analysis has the purpose of discovering the relationship between individual health (capital) and its fundamental determinants, using a picture taken at a given instant.	$h_{ij} = X_{ij}\beta + W_j\beta + SC_{ij}\alpha + \varepsilon_{ij}$, where h_{ij} is a health outcome; X_{ij} is a set of individual-level exogenous variables (e.g., gender, age, family background); W_j is a set of exogenous community characteristics (e.g., pollution, health care supply, crime); SC_{ij} is the set of social capital measures, which could be either at the individual level or at the community level; and ε_{ij} is the	

(Continued)

Table 6.1: (Continued)

Chapter	Name of Measure	Concept	Measure	Rating
			residual unexplained variability of h_{ij}, which contains both unobservable/unavailable determinants and random shocks. The parameters of interest are included in the vector α, which represents the contribution of social capital measures to health.	1
Chapter 8: "Social Capital and Health in Low- and Middle-Income Countries," by Anchorena, Ronconi, and Ozawa	Social Capital and Health in Developed Countries	Social capital is positively correlated with better health outcomes in the developing world, and some studies show that there is a causal relationship. With the exception of trust, which has a larger return in more developed countries, the magnitude of the effects does not appear to vary by the level of economic development.		1
Chapter 9: "Social Capital and Smoking," by Rocco and d'Hombres	Social Capital and Smoking/Health-Related Behaviors	This analysis of the relationship between social capital and smoking, and more generally between social capital and health-related behaviors, has been the only attempt to study a specific pathway through which social capital influences individual health.	To determine whether the impact of bans on smoking prevalence and intensity is larger among individuals with high levels of social capital, the study uses data collected immediately before and immediately after the implementation of smoking bans in public places in Germany between 2007 and 2008.	3

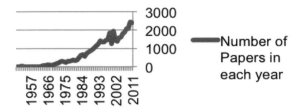

Figure 6.2: "Social Capital and Health." Keyword — Publications per year.
Source: PubMed, NCBI: Medline Index.

seen in the number of publications written every year regarding health, medical care, and mortality listed in three major literature indices: The PubMed Biomedical NCBI Medline Index, the Social Science Citation Index, and the Science Citation Index.

The number of publications with the keywords "social capital AND health" has increased dramatically in all three indexes. The PubMed Medline index shows that in 1951 there were only about 21 items published in the database that matched the *social capital AND health* keyword search. This number has since grown to about 2,500 papers published in 2011 (Figure 6.2). The Social Science Citation Index, which lists publications from 1900 to the present, indicates that 10 papers were published in 1994, while in 2011 that number increased to 205 papers that have been cited 30,577 times, with an average of 1,528 citations per year (Figure 6.3). The Science Citation Index also indicates an upward trend, with only five papers published in 1944 and 140 in 2011. These papers were cited 15,485 times, with an average of 774 citations per year (Figure 6.4).

The keyword search "social capital AND medical care" also indicated an upward incline, as the PubMed Medline index shows a steady increase between 1957 and 1981 and a dramatic spike between 1981 and 2011. In 1957 only two papers were published in the index, but there were 51 in 1981, 121 in 1986, 368 in 1997, and 426 in 2011 (Figure 6.5). The Social Science Citation index also reports an increase in the number of papers published and that these papers were cited 2,726 times, with an average of 151 citations per year (Figure 6.6). The Science Citation index indicated an upward trend as well, with its papers on the subject cited 3,048 times, with an average of 169 citations per year (Figure 6.7).

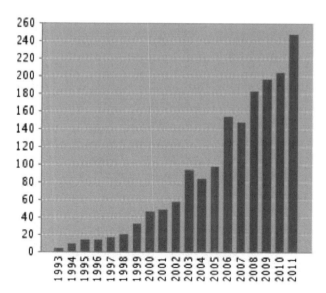

Figure 6.3: "*Social Capital and Health.*" *Keyword Search — Publications per year (SSCI).*
Source: Social Science Citation Index (1900–present).

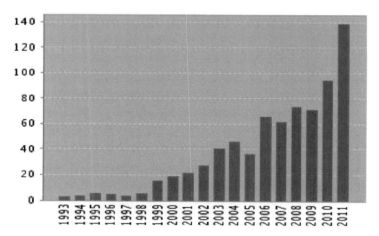

Figure 6.4: "*Social Capital and Health.*" *Keyword Search — Publications per year (SCI).*
Source: Science Citation Index Expanded (1899–Present).

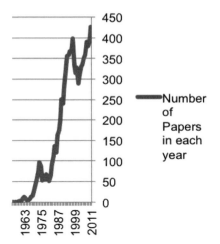

Figure 6.5: "Social Capital and Medical Care." Keyword Search — Number of Publications per year (PubMed).
Source: PubMed, NCBI: Medline Index (1961–2011).

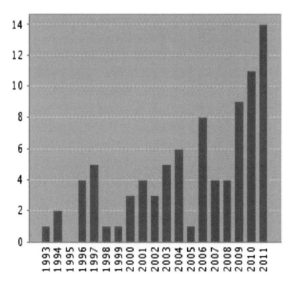

Figure 6.6: "Social Capital and Medical Care." Keyword Search — Number of Publications per year (SSCI).
Source: Social Science Citation Index (1900–2011).

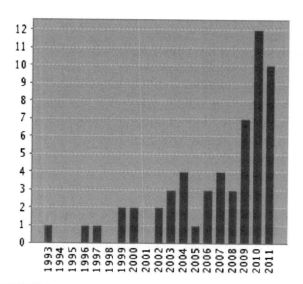

Figure 6.7: "Social Capital and Medical Care." Keyword Search — Publications per year (SCI).
Source: Science Citation Index (1899–2011).

Social capital has also been explored in terms of health outcomes, including mortality, and the number of papers published per year with the keywords "social capital AND mortality" has been on an incline. The PubMed Medline Index shows that, while only two papers with the keywords social capital and mortality were published in 1951, the number increased to 79 papers in 1983 and then dramatically spiked in 1985 with 154 papers. Since 1985 there has been an increasing trend, with 196 papers published in 2011 (Figure 6.8). The Social Science Citation Index shows that, while only three papers were published in 1993, this number rose to 45 papers published in 2011. The index shows that papers on social capital and mortality were cited 13,699 times, with an average of 761 citations per year (Figure 6.9). The Science Citation Index has also seen development and growth in the area of research concerning social capital and its relationship with health, as in 1994 no papers on the subject were published, while 40 papers were published in 2011. These papers have been cited 7,864 times, with an average of 436 citations per year (Figure 6.10).

Clearly, there has been a significant increase in the scholarship regarding health, medical care, and mortality and their relationship to social capital. A variety of academic disciplines, including those in the biomedical, social science,

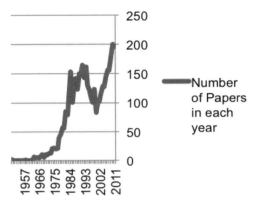

Figure 6.8: "Social Capital and Mortality." Keyword Search — Publications per year (PubMed).

Source: PubMed, NCBI Medline Index (1957–2011).

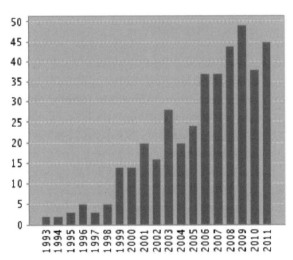

Figure 6.9: "Social Capital and Mortality." Keyword Search — Publications per year (SSCI).

Source: Social Science Citation Index (1993–2011).

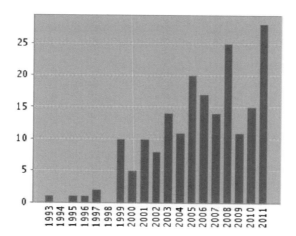

Figure 6.10: "Social Capital and Mortality." Keyword Search — Publications per year (I).
Source: Social Science Citation Index (1993–2011).

and scientific fields, are expanding on early definitions and employing their own definitions using multiple academic contexts. The health and public health outcomes and implications associated with social capital are fostering a modern contribution to this field of research.

International Social Capital

Data from the World Values Survey Questionnaire 2005–2006 can be used to establish the correlation between health and happiness and the relationship between health and happiness and social capital, and these relationships can be used to explore the impact of social capital internationally (Table 6.2). The survey, which includes data from 57 countries, is a global research project that explores people's values and beliefs. Data from the World Values Survey Questionnaire is often employed by researchers, journalists, economists, political scientists, sociologists, and others to extrapolate the differences and similarities in the values of populations around the world.

The World Values Survey Questionnaire 2005–2006 contains 259 questions. For the purpose of this chapter, the following questions on happiness and health and questions that are indicators of social capital, including those on trust,

Table 6.2: Ranking of countries using World Values Survey data.

Country	Health	Happiness	Trust	Friends	Active Membership in Organizations
Malaysia	1	5	52	21	32
Jordan	2	27	31	24	51
Taiwan	3	32	26	28	44
Andorra	4	11	47	8	19
Switzerland	5	7	50	5	7
Canada	6	4	54	2	4
The United States	7	10	48	7	8
New Zealand	7	1	7	48	6
Ghana	9	43	15	40	1
Spain	10	13	45	10	41
South Korea	11	24	34	21	37
Norway	12	2	1	54	21
Argentina	13	23	35	20	40
South Africa	14	44	14	41	16
Sweden	15	3	55	1	23
Uruguay	16	29	29	26	39
Cyprus	17	25	33	22	33
Indonesia	18	9	49	6	10
Thailand	19	12	46	9	20
Australia	20	16	42	13	18
Morocco	21	38	20	34	47
Brazil	22	19	39	16	14
Great Britain	23	8	19	35	12
Italy	24	21	37	18	34
Trinidad and Tobago	25	53	na	51	13
The Netherlands	26	40	na	10	17
Colombia	27	41	17	na	35
France	28	46	12	29	27
Burkina Faso	29	26	32	23	29
Zambia	30	36	22	32	3
Germany	30	51	7	48	28
India	32	15	43	12	10
Turkey	33	20	38	17	52
Iran	34	50	8	47	29
Finland	35	34	24	30	24
Egypt	36	42	16	38	53
Iraq	37	33	25	29	na
Ethiopia	38	47	11	44	15
Mexico	39	39	19	35	9

(Continued)

Table 6.2: (Continued)

Country	Health	Happiness	Trust	Friends	Active Membership in Organizations
Guatemala	40	56	2	53	na
Hong Kong	41	22	36	19	na
Mali	42	35	23	31	2
China	43	18	40	15	43
Chile	44	57	1	54	31
Vietnam	45	6	52	3	25
Slovenia	46	49	9	46	26
Poland	47	17	41	14	42
Bulgaria	48	55	3	52	50
Serbia	49	48	10	45	26
Japan	50	31	16	37	38
Moldova	51	51	7	47	36
Romania	52	37	21	32	42
Peru	53	28	30	24	22
Ukraine	54	30	27	26	45
Georgia	55	45	13	2	54
Russian Federation	56	14	44	33	48
Rwanda	57	54	4	1	5

friendship and membership in organizations, were selected for analysis across all 57 countries:

Happiness

- Question 10: Taking all things together, would you say you are:
  - o Very Happy
  - o Rather happy
  - o Not very happy
  - o Not at all happy

Health

- Question 11: All in all, how good would you describe your state of health these days? Would you say it is:
  - o Very good
  - o Good
  - o Fair

Trust

- Question 23: Generally speaking, would you say that most people can be trusted or that you need to be very careful in dealing with people?

    1. Most people can be trusted
    2. Need to be very careful

Friendship

- Question 5: Friends are

    1. Very important
    2. Rather Important
    3. Not Important
    4. Not at all important

Membership in Organizations Active or Inactive in:

    Question 24: Church or religious organization

    Question 25: Sport or recreational organization

    Question 26: Art, music or educational organization

    Question 27: Labor union

    Question 28: Political party

    Question 29: Environmental organization

    Question 30: Professional association

    Question 31: Humanitarian or charitable organization

    Question 32: Consumer organization

Methodology: Happiness and health calculations and correlations

In order to determine the correlation between happiness and health, questions 10 and 11 were used to rank the 57 countries examined for the survey. For the happiness question, the responses "very happy" and "rather happy" were added for each country, and for the health question the responses "very good" and good" were added for each country. The countries were then ranked based on health (most to least healthy) and happiness (most to least happy). The top 10 countries in regard to health were Malaysia, Jordan, Taiwan, Andorra, Switzerland, Canada, the United States, New Zealand, Ghana, and Spain, and the least healthy country was Rwanda. The top 10 happiest countries were New Zealand, Norway, Sweden,

Canada, Malaysia, the Netherlands, Switzerland, Great Britain, Indonesia, and the United States, and the least happy country was Moldova. The correlation between health and happiness was 0.497.

Methodology: Social capital measures and calculations

The measures of trust, friendship, and membership in organizations were analyzed across the 57 countries, and the correlations between the measures and with health and happiness were calculated. For question 23 regarding trust, there were two possible responses, so countries were ranked based on the percentage of people who responded that "most people can be trusted." For friendship the responses "very important" and "rather important" were added, and countries were ranked based on friendship's being the most important to least important. In regard to membership in organizations, all the responses that indicated that the respondent was active in an organization (for the seven questions on membership) were added, and countries were ranked based on respondents' being the most involved to least involved.

Trust and correlations

The most trusting countries were Norway, Sweden, Finland, Switzerland, China, Vietnam, New Zealand, and Australia. Responses indicated that Trinidad and Tobago were the lowest-ranked in terms of trust. The correlation between trust and health was 0.393, the correlation between trust and happiness was 0.783, the correlation between trust and friendship was 0.814, and the correlation between trust and active membership in organizations was 0.063.

Friendship and correlations

The top ranked countries based on the responses to the question regarding friendship were Rwanda, Georgia, Norway, Finland, Sweden, Turkey, Ethiopia, Great Britain, Switzerland, and the Netherlands. The lowest-ranked was Peru. The correlation between friendship and health was 0.218, that between friendship and happiness was 0.577, that between friendship and trust was 0.814, and that between friendship and membership in organizations was 0.081.

Membership in organizations and correlations

The top ranked countries based on the responses to the seven questions regarding active membership in organizations were Ghana, Mali, Zambia, Canada, Rwanda, New Zealand, Switzerland, the United States and Mexico. The lowest-ranked country was Georgia. The correlation between membership and health was 0.253, that between membership and happiness was 0.157, that between membership and trust was 0.063, and that between membership and friendship was 0.0807.

Summary and Concluding Remarks

Our analysis shows that happiness and health have the strongest correlation (0.50), followed by the correlation between health and trust (0.40). Health and friendship and health and active membership in organizations are similarly correlated (0.21 and 0.25, respectively), and there are significantly strong correlations between happiness and trust, friendship and happiness, and trust and friendship.

Switzerland, Canada, the US, New Zealand, Norway, and Sweden had consistently high rankings, with the countries all ranked in the top twenty for health, happiness, trust, friends, and membership in organizations. (Switzerland was ranked in the top 10 for all categories.) The calculations produced using the World Values Survey Questionnaire 2005–2006 clearly show that there are correlations between social capital measures and health, and this data supports the concept that values used to describe social capital contribute to the well-being of populations.

References

(A)

Averett, S., Argys, L. M. and Kohn, J. 2012. Friends with health benefits: Does individual level social capital improve health? (Working Paper).

Berchet, C., Laporte, A. and Jusot, F. 2012. Immigrant self-rated health and health care utilization in Canada: A casual influence of social capital? (Working Paper).

Berchet, C. and Sirven, N. 2012. Cross-country performance in social integration of older migrants: A European perspective, 1–22. (Working Paper). Health Economics of Ageing and Participation in Society Research Program.

Blanchad, J., Singh, D. and Mignone, J. 2012. Migration, social capital and HIV/AIDS: Understanding the relationship dynamics (Working Paper).

Corman, H., Noonan, K. and Reichman, N. 2012. Effects of postpartum depression on social interactions (Working Paper).

Fiorillo, D. and Sabatini F. 2012. Structural social capital and health in Italy (Working Paper).

Folland, S., Islam, K. M. and Kaarbøe, O. M. 2012. Social capital and types of illness: A look at how its results are achieved (Working Paper).

Gagliardi, C., Rosa, M. D. and Lattanzio, F. 2012. Opportunities for social integration and perceived health status among European older people (Working Paper). National Institute of Health and Science on Aging.

Halla, M. and Zweimuller, M. 2012. The social gradient in the impact of the Chernobyl accident: The case of Austria (Working Paper).

Rocco, L. and d'Hombres, B. 2012. Social capital and smoking (Working Paper).

(B)

Belliveau, M., O'Reilly, C. I. and Wade, J. 1996. Social capital at the top: Effects of social similarity and status on CEO compensation. *The Academy of Management Journal*, 39(6): 1568–1593.

Bourdieu, P. 1986. The forms of capital. In *Handbook of Theory and Research for the Sociology of Education*, ed. Richardson, J., New York: Greenwood, pp. 241–258.

Brown, T. and Scheffler, R. 2008. Social capital, economics, and health: New evidence. *Health Economics, Policy and Law*, 3: 321–331.

Coleman, J. S. 1990. *Foundations of Social Theory*. Cambridge: Harvard University Press, p. 302.

Coleman, J. S. 1988. Social capital in the creation of human capital. *The American Journal of Sociology*, 94, S95–S120.

Friedman, R. and Krackhardt, D. 1997. Social capital and career mobility: A structural theory of lower returns to education for Asian employees. *Journal of Applied Behavioral Science*, 33(3): 316–334.

Fukuyama, F. 1997. *Trust: The Social Virtues and the Creation of Prosperity*. London: Hamish Hamilton.

Glaeser, E. L., Laibson, D. and Sacerdote, B. 2002. An economic approach to social capital. *The Economic Journal*, 112: 437–458.

Grootaert C. and Seralgedin, I. 1998. Defining social capital: An integrating view. In *Social Capital: A Multifaceted Perspective Social*, eds. Dasgupta, P. and Seralgeldin, I., Washington DC: World Bank Publications.

Hannerz, U. 1969. *Soulside: Inquiries into Ghetto Culture and Community*. New York: Columbia.

Jacobs, J. 1961. *The Death and Life of Great American Cities*. New York: Vintage.

Kreuter, M. 1998. Is social capital a mediating structure for effective community-based health promotion? Working paper, Health 2000. Atlanta, GA. (Cited in Easterling *et al.*, 1998).

Lin, N. 1999. Building a network theory of social capital. *Connections*, 22(1): 25–51.

Loury, G. 1977. A dynamic theory of radical income differences. In *Women, Minorities and Employment Discrimination*, eds. Wallace, P. and LeMund, A. Lexington: Lexington Books.

Mignone, J. 2004. Social capital in first nations communities: Conceptual development and instrument validation, Ph.D. Thesis, University of Manitoba.

Moore, S., Daniel, M., Gauvin, L. and Dubè, L. 2009. Not all social capital is good capital. *Health and Place*, 15(4): 1071–1077.

Pennings, J. M, Lee, K and van Witteloostuijn, A. 1998. Human capital social capital and firm survival. *The Academy of Management Journal*, 41(4): 425– 440.

Portes, A. and Sensenbrenner, J. 1993. Embeddedness and immigration: Notes on the social determinants of economic action. *American Journal of Sociology*, 98(6): 1320–1350.

Portes, A. 1998. Social capital: Its origins and applications in modern sociology. *Annual Reviews Sociology,* 24: 1–24

Portes, A. 2000. The two meanings of social capital, *Sociological Forum,* 15(1): 1–12.

Putnam, R. D. 1993. *Making Democracy Work: Civic Traditions in Modern Italy*. Princeton: Princeton University Press.

Putnam, R. D. 2000. *Bowling Alone: The Collapse and Revival of American Community.* New York: Simon & Schuster.

Szreter, S. and Woolcock, M. 2004. Health by association? Social capital, social theory, and the political economy of public health. *International Journal of Epidemiology*, 33: 650–667.

Serageldin, I. and Grootaert, C. 2000. Defining social capital: An integrating view. In *Social Capital: A Multifaceted Perspective*, eds. Dasgupta, P. and Serageldin, I. Washington, D.C.: World Bank Publications.

Sirianni, C, and Friedland, L. 1997. Civic innovation and American democracy. Civic Practices Network.

World Bank. 2011. What is Social Capital? Available at http://go.worldbank.org/ K4LUMW43B0.(accessed on 22 July 2013).

Yamamura, E. 2011. Different effects of social capital on health status among residents: Evidence from modern Japan. *Journal of Socio-Economics* (forthcoming).

Chapter 7

The Empirics of Social Capital and Health

Lorenzo Rocco and Elena Fumagalli

Introduction

The interest in the relationship between social capital and health has risen steadily from both the theoretical and the empirical viewpoint. Social capital has been defined as the glue of society, which has led researchers to naturally hypothesize that individual health could benefit from more collaborative social interactions among friends, neighbors, and the local community. Social capital could produce such an advantage to health through several pathways: Social capital could favor the formation of informal networks and safety nets that provide mutual insurance to their members in case of health shocks (Murgai *et al.*, 2002); increase the political strength of a community, making it easier to obtain more and better public goods and more generous social welfare programs (Kawachi *et al.*, 1997); reduce moral hazard in the relationship between local health providers and patients (Laporte *et al.*, 2008); shield people against the stress of uncertainty (Wilkinson, 1996); and expand the informational resources that are available to individuals, allowing for a faster and more intense circulation of information about the quality of local health care services (Scheffler and Brown, 2008). Recent evidence (Brown *et al.*, 2011; Brown *et al.*, 2006) also suggests that social capital contributes to reducing smoking, as more cohesive societies are more effective at enforcing anti-smoking norms and regulations (see d'Hombres and Rocco's chapter in this book, Chapter 9).

These arguments are compelling enough to justify the extensive research that has been produced, especially in the last few years, and has resulted in many papers empirically assessing the influence of both collective and individual social capital. These papers consider several health outcomes and many different countries, covering all the populated continents with the possible exception of

Africa. Reduced-form models have been usually estimated. Such models focus on whether there is any significant association between social capital and health, but by their own nature, they do not distinguish among the possible mechanisms through which social capital influences health.

In this chapter, we discuss the empirical literature on social capital and health and analyze a number of difficulties that emerge in empirical analyses and that must be addressed or taken into account in order to produce credible estimates. The major empirical problem is essentially related to the endogeneity of social capital, denounced by Durlauf (2002) and Durlauf and Fafchaps (2005) and now widely recognized.[7] We then discuss endogeneity in the framework of the "health reduced form model" — that is, the model that links health to its fundamental determinants. This framework has been almost unanimously adopted in the literature on social capital and health. We distinguish among the three major sources of endogeneity — reverse causation, omitted variables and measurement errors — and mention the specific reasons why social capital should be viewed as endogenous. Then within the framework of the "health reduced form model," we consider a specific problem that can emerge when individual and community social capital are simultaneously included in the model. The following section moves to the peer effects framework adopted by Durlauf (2002) in his critique of the "empirics of social capital." Durlauf points out that, when social capital is considered a characteristic of peers, it is difficult to isolate the effect of social capital from the effect of peers and other correlated factors. We first analyze Durlauf's argument and then relate Durlauf's setting to the health reduced-form model.

---

[7]A variable is said to be endogenous when there are conceptual reasons that suggest a correlation between the variable and the error term of the empirical equation under estimation. Symmetrically, a variable is exogenous if it is uncorrelated with the error term. Some authors adopt a stricter definition of endogeneity and define it as the correlation emerging when social capital is endogenously and jointly determined with the health outcome within the model. For instance, Durlauf (2002) distinguishes between two causes of correlation, naming "exchangeability of the error terms" the correlation that is due to omitted variables, and "endogeneity" the correlation arising by the endogenous determination of social capital. Formally, Durlauf's (2002) exchangeability definition is "conditional on all available information, the probability of observing a given vector of error realizations (one each observation) is equal to the probability of observing any permutation of the previous vector. This general property implies that errors are i.i.d. conditional to the included regressors, which in turn implies conditional independence of the error term."

Comprehensive solutions or "golden rules" to overcome these problems do not exist, so specific estimation strategies have to be devised each time by balancing the relative advantages and drawbacks of alternative estimation techniques in the specific context of analysis. Nevertheless, some guidance can be found in the literature. We reviewed the recent empirical literature on the adopted estimation strategies in order to provide a useful case list to compare with the concrete situation one is considering and to provide an initial benchmark. We then discuss the empirical literature produced in the last five years, distinguishing among studies that seek to estimate causal effects and studies that look for associations. We also mention a small, recent body of literature that examines the inverse relationship — that is, the influence of health on individual social capital — and provide a summary of findings, produced by means of experimental methods, on the informative content of "generalized trust," one of the most commonly used measures of social capital.

We next perform a simple Monte Carlo experiment in order to provide some sense, in a controlled environment, of the magnitude of the bias that could plague estimates when a particular source of endogeneity is not adequately treated. More specifically, we look at the problem of unobservable community factors correlated with individual social capital. In the final section, we conclude.

Endogeneity in the Health Reduced-Form Model

The literature on the determinants of health is based on the theoretical model proposed by Grossman in 1972. Grossman's dynamic model is one in which individuals accumulate health capital over time, just as they do with financial and human capital: They dispose of a technology, called a "health production function," that transforms inputs in health. Inputs include medical services, lifestyles, and working and housing conditions. At each point in time, utility-maximizing individuals will have accumulated a given amount of health capital according to the optimal investment plan they have defined at the beginning of the period. As the paths of accumulation each individual adopts are optimal, differences among individuals' health conditions depend only on differences in their "initial conditions," such as preferences, endowments (earning ability, family background, genetic endowment) and the constraints they have faced during their life (environmental, economic, and social factors). We name these initial conditions the fundamental determinants of individual health that influence the decisions of individual investment in health and lifestyle but which are beyond individual control. From this perspective, the health condition of two individuals who are perfectly alike in terms of their fundamental determinants can differ only because of random shocks since the optimal path of accumulation is otherwise identical. From a theoretical perspective, health is the unique endogenous variable since it is the outcome of the optimization process, while the fundamental causes are the exogenously given parameters and constraints of the problem.

Grounded on Grossman's model, the empirical analysis has one important purpose: That of discovering the relationship between individual health (capital) and its fundamental determinants, taking a picture at a given instant. At that time, the observed amount of individual health capital depends on the stage of the accumulation process at which each individual stands and, of course, on the level of the fundamental determinants, which is individual-specific.

Operationally, a health reduced-form model is defined as one where individual health is "regressed" on a battery more or less complete of fundamental determinants. In the health reduced-form model, the process of health capital accumulation and other important issues, such as the demand function of medical services, remain in the background; the focus is entirely on the "comparative statics" that map fundamental determinants into optimal outcomes of the health accumulation process.

For illustration purposes we distinguish social capital from all other fundamental determinants and write the health reduced-form model as:

$$h_{ij} = X_{ij}\beta + W_j\delta + SC_{ij}\alpha + \varepsilon_{ij} \tag{7.1}$$

where h_{ij} is a health outcome, X_{ij} is a set of individual-level exogenous variables (e.g., gender, age, family background), W_j is a set of exogenous community characteristics (e.g., pollution, health care supply, crime), and SC_{ij} is the set of social capital measures, which could be either at the individual level or at the community level. Finally, ε_{ij} represents the residual unexplained variability of h_{ij}, which contains both unobservable/unavailable determinants and random shocks. The parameters of interest are included in the vector α, which represents the contribution of social capital measures to health.

Although any fundamental determinant is, by definition, exogenous from the theoretical viewpoint, nothing prevents that the actual regressors included in (7.1), and especially so social capital, are correlated with the error term. From the econometric viewpoint, nothing prevents social capital from being endogenous. Social capital could be endogenous, for instance, if some relevant community characteristics were omitted from Eq. (7.1). As omitted variables would be absorbed into the error term, a correlation between the residual itself and social capital would arise almost mechanically. Therefore, paradoxically, a fundamental determinant can simultaneously be exogenous from the theoretical viewpoint and endogenous from the empirical perspective.[8]

Endogeneity makes the empirical identification[9] of the parameter of interest, α, difficult. Formally, endogeneity is stated as

$$E(SC_{ij}\varepsilon_{ij}|X_{ij},\ {}^{\cdot}W_j) \neq 0 \qquad (7.2)$$

Under condition (7.2) the OLS estimated parameter $\tilde{a}$ would be biased and inconsistent. The sign and the size of the bias $\tilde{a} - \alpha$ is generally unpredictable and can be so large that it leads to largely misleading conclusions.

Endogeneity has many causes, but they are generally classified into three broad categories: Reverse causation, omitted variables, and measurement errors, each of which we discuss below.

Reverse causation

Reverse causation refers to the possibility that the dependent variable influences the supposed explanatory variable, creating a feedback or circular relationship. Reverse causation generates a mechanical correlation between the explanatory variable and the error term, even if the residual includes only purely random noise.

In social capital and health analysis, it is not unreasonable to suspect that individual health might have a role in determining individual social capital. For instance, healthier people could have more opportunities for social interaction and social exchange and participate more easily in social organizations, so they would ultimately accumulate more social capital.

As Guiso *et al.* (2008a) suggest, social capital can be defined as the individual's belief about the willingness of other people to cooperate. Although the initial endowment of social capital (i.e., prior beliefs) is transmitted by parents, social

---

[8]These multiple meanings of the words "exogenous" and "endogenous," depending on the perspective one adopts, can easily cause confusion and misunderstanding between theorists and empiricists, and between economists and scientists of other disciplines.

[9]Identification refers to the possibility of recovering directly or indirectly an *unbiased* estimate of α from the parameters estimated in the model.

capital is continuously updated by means of social interactions.[10] If healthier people have more intense social interactions that allow them to acquire better information about others' willingness to cooperate, they will acquire more information and be able to form better predictions compared to people in poorer health. Therefore, the current level of social capital depends on current and past health conditions.

Suppose that parents transfer pessimistic beliefs[11] to their sons to protect them from the risk of being exploited by other people (Guiso *et al.*, 2008a). In that case, the more intense social interactions allowed by better health conditions will produce more "socially favorable" beliefs, thus increasing individual social capital. Since both the effect of health on social capital and the effect of the residual on health are positive, there will be a *positive* correlation between social capital and ε_{ij}.

To see how OLS estimates react in this case, suppose that ε_{ij} is decomposed into two parts, one correlated with social capital and one orthogonal (formally, this amounts to projecting ε_{ij} on SC_{ij}). Write $\varepsilon_{ij} = \lambda SC_{ij} + \phi_{ij}$, where λ is a positive parameter that captures the correlation between social capital and the residual. By substituting ε_{ij} in Eq. (7.1), we obtain

$$h_{ij} = X_{ij}\beta + W_j\delta + (\alpha + \lambda)SC_{ij} + \phi_{ij} \tag{7.3}$$

Equation (7.3), not Eq. (7.1), is what will be estimated by OLS in practice. Therefore, the estimated parameter of social capital will be $(\alpha + \lambda)$ instead of the structural true parameter α. Thus, in this particular example, OLS estimates will be biased upward because of the feedback effect (λ) from health to social capital, which offers a too-optimistic indication about the beneficial role of social capital on health.

The direction of the bias depends on the sign of λ, that is, on the sign of the feedback effect from health to social capital.

Omitted variables

The second reason for a correlation between an explanatory variable and the error term is the so-called "omitted variable problem," which refers to a situation in which one or more relevant explanatory variables, correlated with the included

---

[10]Accordingly, only the initial endowment transmitted by parents is a fundamental determinant of health.

[11]Parents transmit distorted beliefs to their sons.

explanatory variable of interest, are omitted from the model specification either by mistake or because they are unavailable.

To illustrate, suppose that the correctly specified model is (7.1), but that, because of lack of data, we estimate instead:

$$h_{ij} = X_{ij}\beta + SC_{ij}\alpha + \eta_{ij} \qquad (7.1')$$

where community level variables W_j have been omitted. The residual η_{ij} then includes the omitted variables so that $\eta_{ij} = W_j\delta + \varepsilon_{ij}$. If community-level variables were correlated with social capital, then their omission would certainly alter the estimated parameter of social capital. Decompose now W_j into two parts, one positively correlated and one orthogonal to social capital, and write $W_j = \lambda SC_{ij} + \phi_{ij}$. Thus, we can rewrite (7.1') as

$$h_{ij} = X_{ij}\beta + (\alpha + \delta\lambda)SC_{ij} + (\delta\phi_{ij} + \varepsilon_{ij})$$

Suppose $\delta > 0$ and $corr(W_j, SC_{ij}) > 0$ such that $\lambda > 0$. Under these hypotheses, the omission of community-level variables will induce an upward bias in the estimated effect of social capital. The sign of the bias will depend on the sign of the correlation between social capital and the omitted variables and on the sign of the omitted variable's effect on health. While the omitted variable problem can sometimes be solved by adding controls to the model, in many cases important variables are omitted because they are simply unobservable. For instance, social capital is likely to be correlated with individual preferences, which are typically unavailable to the researcher. This correlation arises because both the initial social capital endowment and many preference and psychological traits are transmitted and partly shaped by parents (Tabellini, 2010; Bisin and Verdier, 2010; Guiso *et al.*, 2008a). For instance, more risk-averse parents could transmit high risk aversion to their children, along with more pessimistic beliefs about other people's willingness to cooperate. If such risk-averse people were unwilling to take health risks, this situation would create a spurious *negative* correlation between social capital and health, independent of whether social capital does influence health.

Similarly, people with high time discount rates could have more incentive than others to undertake opportunistic behaviors in repeated interactions, in so doing accumulating less social capital. At the same time they could be more indulgent towards unhealthy lifestyles, as they heavily discount the associated future losses. This pattern of behavior would then generate a spurious *positive* correlation between social capital and health. Analogous reasoning could be generated for other traits or individual preferences. Generally speaking, the omission of any preference or trait will produce biases in the OLS estimate of social capital's effect on health, the direction of which is difficult to determine *ex ante*.

In addition, the correlation between social capital and the residual that is due to processes of self-selection or self-sorting are ultimately a problem of omitted variables. Individuals who are rich in social capital might tend to associate with people who are equally rich in social capital, given that individuals tend to choose their reference group or their social community. At the extreme, they could also choose their residence by taking into account the level of social capital in the community they plan to join. If social capital is correlated with other individual or community characteristics that influence individual health, it would be difficult to distinguish the effect of the former from that of the latter.

Measurement errors

A third cause of endogeneity is the presence of measurement errors in one or more explanatory variables. Such measurement errors occur when some variables are unavailable and are replaced by proxies or when some variables are affected by mis-reporting.

Social capital indicators are typically proxies, imperfect indices of social capital affected by a non negligible error. Social capital indicators often consist of self-reported beliefs or self-reported membership in social organizations, where either imperfect recall or the desire to please or impress the interviewer can play a role. Error-in-variable mechanically produces a correlation between the included measure of social capital and the error term. When the measurement error is normally distributed and orthogonal to the correct level of social capital (classical error-in-variable), the coefficient of social capital is likely to be downward biased.[12] Non classical errors could bias estimates in either direction. (See Wooldridge, 2002, Chapter 4.4 for a detailed discussion.)

Furthermore, when both social capital and health are self-reported variables collected during the same interview, contingent psychological conditions, optimism, or depression could bias both reports in the same direction, thus creating an artificial positive correlation between the two. Fujiwara and Kawachi (2008) called such a situation "common method bias." Reporting heterogeneity of the type "cut-point shift" (Lindeboom and van Doorslaer, 2004) can also bias the results. The only

---

[12]It is certainly so only in univariate regressions.

option for overcoming these difficulties is to adopt more objective measures of health. In the few studies in which more closely objective measures of health are used along with individual social capital (Hyppa *et al.*, 2007; Borgonovi, 2010), the positive association between social capital and health remains.

Individual and Community Social Capital Together

Another empirical problem arises when both individual-level social capital (ISC) and community-level social capital (CSC) are included in the model, and the latter is determined as the average of ISC at the community level. Consider the following simplified version of Eq. (7.1):

$$h_{ij} = \alpha_0 + \alpha_1 ISC_{ij} + \alpha_2 CSC_j + \varepsilon_{ij} \qquad (7.1'')$$

where we distinguish between ISC and CSC. Define $CSC_j = \frac{1}{N_j} \sum_{i=1}^{N_j} ISC_{ij}$, that is, suppose that CSC in community j is the average of ISC among all residents of community j. Acemoglu and Angrist (2001) note that there is a mechanical link between OLS estimates of α_1 and α_2 that renders identification of the structural parameters impossible. To see this, let ρ_1 be the OLS estimate of a bivariate regression of h_{ij} on ISC_{ij} alone, and let ρ_2 be the coefficient of a bivariate regression of h_{ij} on CSC_j alone. Note also that the latter is equivalent to the 2SLS estimate of a bivariate regression of h_{ij} on ISC_{ij}, where ISC_{ij} is instrumented by a full set of community dummies. Because of this equivalence, OLS estimates of (7.1'') can be written as $\alpha_1 = \rho_2 + \varphi(\rho_1 - \rho_2)$ and $\alpha_2 = -\varphi(\rho_1 - \rho_2)$, where $\varphi = \frac{1}{1-R^2} > 1$, and R^2 is the first-stage R^2 when community dummies are used as instruments for ISC_{ij}. If for any reason the OLS and the 2SLS estimates of the bivariate regression of h_{ij} on ISC_{ij} differed, then certainly we would obtain a nonzero coefficient of CSC_j, even if no association actually existed. Suppose, for instance, that the 2SLS estimate corrects for measurement error in ISC_{ij} thus eliminating the downward bias. Then certainly $\rho_2 > \rho_1$, making $\alpha_2 > 0$. If, instead, the 2SLS corrects for a positive correlation with relevant omitted variables, then $\rho_2 < \rho_1$ and $\alpha_2 < 0$. Finally, if ISC were exogenous and community dummies were appropriate instruments, then $\rho_2 = \rho_1$ as OLS and 2SLS would coincide, and $\alpha_2 = 0$.[13] Breaking the link between α_1 and α_2 is possible by means of a sophisticated

---

[13]This is an unlikely case, as community dummies are typically not proper instruments for ISC.

IV strategy in which both ISC_{ij} and CSC_j are considered endogenous and instrumented.[14]

Therefore, studies that include both ISC and CSC risk providing inaccurate conclusions about the effects of CSC. However, this result depends on CSC's being defined as the average of ISC on the entire community. There are two ways out of this conundrum: First, alternative indicators of ISC and CSC, such as, generalized trust and the Petris Index, can be used. Second, if CSC is nonetheless defined as an average of ISC, partially overlapping communities should be used. Communities are partially overlapping when the community of individual i does not perfectly coincide with the community of at least one member of individual i's community (De Giorgi et al., 2010). Rocco et al. (2013) offer an example of partially overlapping communities by defining individual i's community as the residents in region i whose age does not differ from that of i by more than 10 years.[15]

Peer Effects and Social Capital

In this section we leave for a moment the health reduced-form model to discuss a more structural way of analyzing the influence of social capital on health by looking at the peer effects framework, a setting in which individual health-related behaviors depend on peers' health behaviors. Here, the role of social capital is that of influencing and modifying such inter-dependence between individual actions. Differently from the health reduced form model, whose purpose is that of discovering the link between general health and its fundamental determinants, we are now looking more closely at specific decisions that are taken at a given point in time and enter as inputs into the health production function. For instance, adopting the peer effects framework is the natural approach if we want to analyze

---

[14]The choice of instruments should respect the following condition: suppose Z is an appropriate instrument for CSC_j. Then an appropriate instrument T for ISC_{ij} should be such that the IV effect of ISC_{ij} on health, computed by the Wald formula, coincides with the effect of ISC_{ij} on health (purged of the CSC effect) when ISC_{ij} is instrumented by Z, again computed by the Wald formula. The intuition is essentially that IV estimates capture LATE effects, and the subset of individuals treated by T should be the roughly the same as the subset of individuals treated by Z. (See Acemoglu and Angrist, 2001, for additional details.)

[15]In this case the average social capital in individual i's community does not coincide either with the average social capital at the regional level or with the average social capital of the residents who are the same age as individual i.

smoking, drinking, risky sex, or the willingness to have a medical screening (or, more in generally, medical utilization), where social interaction plays an important role.[16]

We initially discuss the identification problems that emerge in the peer effects framework, adapting the seminal works of Durlauf (2002) and the subsequent Durlauf and Fafchamps (2005)[17] to our context. Durlauf suggests that social capital be treated as a peer characteristic that has an autonomous influence on individual actions in addition to the effect of peers' behavior.[18] Next, we discuss how peer effects can be accounted for in the health reduced-form model.

Identification in the peer effects framework

As Mansky (1993) defines in the most general specification of the problem, peer effects are composed of (a) an *endogenous* component (how peers' behavior affects individual behavior), (b) a *contextual* component (how the exogenous characteristics of peers affect individual behavior), and (c) a *correlated* component (how third variables, such as environmental factors, affect both individual and peer behavior).

Consider the following equation:

$$Y_{ij} = \beta_0 + \beta_1 \overline{Y}_j + \beta_2 \overline{SC}_j + \beta_3 SC_{ij} + \beta_4 \overline{W}_j + \beta_{51} W_{ij} + \beta_{52} X_{ij} + \beta_6 Z_j + \varepsilon_{ij}$$

$$(7.4)$$

and suppose that Y_{ij} is the health behavior under consideration, such as, whether a person goes for a medical screening for a certain disease; $\overline{Y}_j$ is the average of Y at the community level (supposed for simplicity to coincide with individual i's reference group); SC_{ij} is ISC in community j; $\overline{SC}_j$ is CSC, computed again as an average of ISC; W_{ij} and X_{ij} are relevant individual characteristics, such as education, family background, and income; $\overline{W}_j$ is the community average of the set W_{ij}; and Z_j are environmental factors that influence the choices of all residents in community j, such as the availability of medical centers or the price

---

[16]In the literature, the peer effects setting has been largely employed to analyze smoking, where peers' influence has been found to be an important driver.

[17]These studies discuss the empirics of social capital in general and do not explicitly look at the role of social capital on health.

[18]We start by discussing Durlauf's simplest setting, where social capital is assumed to be exogenous.

of a medical screening, and this makes the behaviors of all residents correlated. As Durlauf (2002) suggests, CSC is considered a contextual factor. Here, we have also included ISC as an individual characteristic for the sake of generality. The critical assumption is that the community averages of X_{ij} can be excluded from Eq. (7.4) — that is, these averages do not have an autonomous effect on Y_{ij}. This restriction is necessary if separate identifications of the endogenous, contextual, and correlated effects are to be achieved. Parameter β_1, which is associated with $\overline{Y}_j$, measures the effect of peers' behavior on individual behavior, so it is the endogenous peer effect. Parameters β_2 and β_4, which are associated with $\overline{SC}_j$ and $\overline{W}_j$, measure contextual peer effects. Finally β_6, the coefficient of Z_j, measures correlated effects.

Identification of all the structural parameters of Eq. (7.4) is made difficult by the presence of $\overline{Y}_j$. Indeed, to be consistent with this specification, model (7.4) as well must determine the health behavior of each peer and therefore, the average peer behavior should be obtained by averaging Eq. (7.4) over all the individuals in the peer group. This process implies a strong correlation — close to perfect multi-collinearity — between $\overline{Y}_j$ and the contextual and correlated factors included in Eq. (7.4), which could prevent identification.[19] Furthermore, a direct estimation of a simplified version of Eq. (7.4), in which contextual and correlated factors are removed, would yield $\beta_1 = 1$, as Angrist and Pischke (2008, p. 195) show.[20]

The first step to obtaining an operational equation to estimate is computing the community average of (7.4), which is solved for $\overline{Y}_j$ to get

$$\overline{Y}_j = \frac{\beta_0}{1 - \beta_1} + \frac{\beta_2 + \beta_3}{1 - \beta_1}\overline{SC}_j + \frac{\beta_4 + \beta_{51}}{1 - \beta_1}\overline{W}_j + \frac{\beta_{52}}{1 - \beta_1}\overline{X}_j + \frac{\beta_6}{1 - \beta_1}Z_j \tag{7.5}$$

Next, by substituting (7.5) back into (7.4), we get the equilibrium condition

$$Y_{ij} = \frac{\beta_0}{1 - \beta_1} + \frac{\beta_2 + \beta_1\beta_3}{1 - \beta_1}\overline{SC}_j + \beta_3 SC_{ij} + \frac{\beta_4 + \beta_1\beta_{51}}{1 - \beta_1}\overline{W}_j$$
$$+ \beta_{51} W_{ij} + \frac{\beta_1\beta_{52}}{1 - \beta_1}\overline{X}_j + \beta_{52} X_{ij} + \frac{\beta_6}{1 - \beta_1}Z_j + \varepsilon_{ij} \tag{7.6}$$

which can now be estimated by OLS.

---

[19]Brock and Durlauf (2001) show that the identification problems of the linear-in-mean model (7.4), which prevents simultaneous identification of endogenous, contextual, and correlated effects because of multi-collinearity, disappear in (nonlinear) discrete choice models, where identification by functional form naturally arises. In these models the average outcome is not linearly related to other community averages.

[20]Partially overlapped groups are sufficient to resolve this problem.

Durlauf (2002) proves that in Eq. (7.6) all structural parameters can be recovered from the OLS estimates, thanks to the assumption that the set X_{ij} of individual characteristics distinct from W_{ij} is non-empty. (This is the essence of Proposition 1 in Durlauf, 2002, p. F466.) Indeed, from the reduced form parameters associated with $\overline{X}_j$ and X_{ij}, we obtain the endogenous peer effect β_1. Next, by knowing β_1 and by using the coefficients of $\overline{SC}_j$ and SC_{ij}, we derive β_2 as the contextual effect of CSC. Finally, by knowing β_1, we recover the correlated effect from the coefficient of Z_j. If, instead, the set X_{ij} is empty — that is, if the community averages of *all* individual characteristics, without exclusions, have direct influence on individual health behavior — then endogenous, contextual, and correlated effects could not be separately identified. There must be good reasons to justify this restriction.[21]

If identification were not possible, perhaps because there were no sensible restrictions to make, the reduced-form parameters of Eq. (7.6) could still be informative. These parameters capture the total effect of the included variables on individual behavior, which total effect is the combination of the direct effects specified in Eq. (7.4) (also called partial effect) and the possible indirect effects that operate through social interaction. For instance, provided that both CSC and ISC tend to encourage prevention, as suggested in the literature, if $0 < \beta_1 < 1$, then the total effect of CSC will have the same sign of the partial effect and will be larger. Thus, the total effect can provide valuable indications when identification of the partial effect fails.

However, in our specification, looking at the total effect of CSC could lead to incorrect conclusions. Given that we assume an autonomous effect of ISC that is in addition to CSC (i.e., given that β_3 is nonzero), the total effect of CSC could be nonzero also if its partial (contextual) effect β_2 is null. Therefore, in the absence of proper identification of the structural parameters, we could conclude that CSC is relevant even if only ISC matters in reality.

Whether the total or the partial effect is more policy-relevant is also debatable. We believe that, in many circumstances, the total effect of social capital is more relevant, as it accounts for the full influence of the variable; however, as we have just seen, the total effect might also be misleading. A final answer will depend

---

[21] Similar restrictions must be assumed if social capital is supposed to be jointly determined with health. We refer to Durlaf (2002) for details.

on the particular model the researcher is considering and on the purpose of the analysis he or she is conducting.

Peer effects in the health reduced-form model

Since peer effects contribute to the health accumulation process, one expects that the health reduced-form model implicitly accounts for them. It is worth investigating whether this is actually the case and how the health reduced-form model should be specified in order to make it capture the influence of peers. Anticipating the result of this analysis, we find that the health reduced form-model accounts for the influence of peers if (exogenous) peers' characteristics are included in the model.

Consider a very stylized model in which individuals derive utility from their own behavior Y_{ij}, from peer behavior $\overline{Y}_j$, and from consumption C. Suppose also that individuals have a technology that creates lifecycle consumption from their health capital. Finally, suppose that the production of health capital is negatively influenced by both individual and peer behavior[22] and that it depends on the fundamental determinants of health X_{ij}, which also include social capital; that is, $h_{ij} = H(Y_{ij}, \overline{Y}_j, X_{ij})$. Therefore, individuals face a trade-off when they optimally choose their level of Y_{ij}, because Y_{ij} gives them pleasure but reduces lifecycle consumption. The optimal choice will be a function of peer behavior $\overline{Y}_j$ and the fundamental determinants of health, $Y_{ij}^* = f(\overline{Y}_j, X_{ij})$. This is the theoretical counterpart of Eq. (7.4). Now compute the equilibrium level of $\overline{Y}_j$ in community j by applying a Nash-equilibrium-type argument. The (average) equilibrium level $\overline{Y}_j^*$ can be approximated[23] by a function of the average fundamental determinants $\overline{X}_j$. Therefore, at equilibrium, individual Y_{ij} can be written as $Y_{ij}^* = g(\overline{X}_j, X_{ij})$, a function of only individual and community fundamental determinants of health. Substituting this expression into the health production function, we have

$$h_{ij}^* = H(Y_{ij}^*, \overline{Y}_j^*, X_{ij}) = h(X_{ij}, \overline{X}_j) \tag{7.7}$$

which is a function of only individual and community fundamental determinants. Equation (7.7) is the health reduced-form model, where the average peer

---

[22]This would be the case for, for example, smoking or drinking. Regarding medical use, we have an initial disutility but a positive effect on health.

[23]More precisely, it would be a function of the complete vector of individual fundamental determinants $[X_{1j}, X_{2j}, \ldots, X_{Nj}]$.

characteristics are controlled for. Therefore, if it is suitably specified, a health reduced-form model will account also for peer effects. However, model (7.7) falls under the situation described in subsection 'Individual and community social, capital together' (p. 101), so complete identification of the effect of individual and peers' fundamental determinants can be achieved only if the groups of peers partially overlap.

The empirical estimation of function (7.7) yields the total effect of the fundamental determinants on equilibrium health. It is not possible to distinguish between direct and indirect — throughout interaction — effects, which looks to be a minor drawback, at least with regards to social capital.

Empirical Strategies Adopted in the Literature

The empirical issues discussed in the three preceding sections should indicate the importance of taking care in estimating the effect of social capital on individual health. Identification of causal effects is difficult, and suitable estimation strategies must be adopted. Looking at simple associations can be misleading, as estimates can be severely biased and, in extreme cases, can have an incorrect sign.

There is no universal recipe that can solve at once all identification problems in all circumstances. Rather, each specific context and each specific analysis requires a specific solution. Manipulating the model or finding less direct ways of addressing the problem sometimes simplifies the quest for identification.

Instrumental variable (IV) estimators are widely considered the leading technique against endogeneity because they are always effective, regardless of the cause of endogeneity. In practice, though, IV requirements are so strict that, in many cases, finding appropriate instruments is exceedingly difficult. In particular, the requirement most difficult to meet is that of exogeneity of the instrument, which requires that instruments be uncorrelated with the regression residual, whatever components the residual might include (e.g., omitted variables at any level, measurement errors, random noise). Examples of instruments that are widely considered acceptable are based on reforms, natural experiments, policy interventions, and shocks, the last of which exploit the variation induced by clearly external-to-the-model interventions. It is no surprise that, in many cases, either these interventions do not exist or there is inadequate information about them. In regard to social capital, the availability of instruments of this type seems particularly unlikely.

When endogenity is due to reverse causation or measurement error, an IV analysis is the only way out. When the principal cause of endogenity is the presence of omitted constant individual or community characteristics, fixed-effect estimators can be used as an alternative to IV because, by construction, they exploit only the variation within individuals or communities to achieve identification, neglecting the variation between individuals and communities, where omitted variables play their role. However, lacking a universal solution to endogeneity, we believe that studying the solutions proposed in the literature could be a good starting point from which to enrich each one's toolbox. In the remaining part of this section, we analyze the recent literature on social capital and health.

Especially in the last decade, the number of papers that have estimated the association between social capital and health has grown significantly, especially in public health journals and multidisciplinary journals, although not so much in economic journals. Several authors (Cooper *et al.*, 1999; Lochner *et al.*, 1999; Macinko and Starfield, 2001; and Muntaner *et al.*, 2001) have reviewed the empirical literature on social capital and health — a very complete survey is compiled by Islam *et al.* (2006a) — but most of the published papers point to associations and only a few seek to identify the causal effect of social capital on health.

We focus on this aspect of social capital and pursued an approach as comprehensive as possible in terms of the criteria for inclusion in our search. Nonetheless, taking into account both published and un-published articles, we found only 12 papers. We organized the key elements of their content in Table 7.1, where we report which data were used, the indicators of social capital and health that were adopted, the estimation technique adopted, and the main results. A general discussion of these contributions is included in subsection 'Causal effects' (p. 109).

For the sake of completeness, we also reviewed a sample of the recently published papers that examine associations. Taking over where Islam (2006a) left off, we reviewed a set of 24 papers published in peer-reviewed journals from 2006 to 2011 that we judged as relevant either for methodological reasons or for the data used. Most of these papers adopt multi-level analysis. A detailed review of the contents is organized in Table 7.2, whose layout parallels that of Table 7.1. We did not attempt to offer a comprehensive discussion of all the published papers, as many differ relatively little from a methodological perspective. The subsection 'Associations' (p. 119) provides a general discussion that focuses on multi-level analysis. To help the reader who is willing to approach the empirical analysis,

Table 7.3 includes a schematic description of the characteristics of the datasets most frequently used that report information on both social capital and health.

In the following subsection 'Causal effects', we spend a few words on a stream of the literature that focuses on the opposite relationship — that is, the relationship that moves from health to social capital. This stream of literature appeared only recently, but we believe it will attract considerable interest in the near future. Finally, we review the literature on the ability of trust questions collected in surveys to predict real behavior in the laboratory and in the real world.

Surprisingly, we have not found any paper which considers the role of social capital in the peer effects framework and properly looks at the identification problems. Some common features have emerged from the review. Most studies distinguish between ISC and CSC where generalized trust and participation to voluntary social organizations are often adopted as indicators of ISC while the average of ISC indicators at the community level are considered measures of CSC. In relatively few contributions alternative indicators are employed, such as voting participation or the Petris Index at the community level. Turning to health, most papers use the widely available self-reported health and only few exceptions adopt more objective health indicators. Overall, social capital is always found to be positively associated with individual health, and especially so with regards to ISC.

Causal effects

Only a few studies have attempted to identify the causal effects of social capital. Three approaches have been followed, the most common of which uses IVs. Two papers have adopted multiple equation models and two other papers some kind of fixed effects (Table 7.1).

IVs require using exogenous sources of variation to achieve identification, although finding appropriate instruments is far from trivial. Besides the relatively easy requirement of relevance — that is, a strong correlation between the instrument and the supposed endogenous social capital variables — instruments must be exogenous, that is, uncorrelated with the error term, condition on the remaining exogenous regressors. One implication of exogeneity is the so-called exclusion restriction, which requires that instruments must have no direct effect on the dependent variable (health) beyond the effect mediated by social capital.

There are no proper tests for the exogeneity/exclusion restriction, so it must be carefully motivated. The use of over-identification tests *à la* Sargan-Hansen

Table 7.1: Selected recent studies that seek a causal relationship between social capital and health.

Reference	Country/Dataset/ Year	Social Capital Indicators	Health Outcomes	Method	Results
Brown et al., 2011	US, California Tobacco Survey, 1999, 2002	At the community level only. Petris Index computed at the county level	Smoking (number of cigarettes)	Instrumental variables estimator. Community social capital and cigarette price are considered endogenous variables (prices are endogenous because of measurement errors). Instrumental variables are weather characteristics at the county level (maximum temperatures, minimum temperatures, maximum wind speed, and maximum precipitation) and indices of racial/ethnic diversity.	Social capital significantly reduces both smoking participation and the number of cigarettes smoked.
d'Hombres et al., 2010	8 former soviet republics, Living Conditions, Lifestyles and Health, 2001	At the individual level, generalized trust, membership in voluntary organizations, social isolation	Self-reported health	Instrumental variable linear probability model, with and without community fixed effects. Instruments are indices of community heterogeneity (religion, education and income) and averages of social capital indicators at the community level. Communities are defined as settlements, according to the LLH definition.	Trust and social isolation are statistically significant determinants of health; no effect of membership.

(Continued)

Table 7.1: (*Continued*)

Reference	Country/Dataset/ Year	Social Capital Indicators	Health Outcomes	Method	Results
Deri, 2005	Canada, National Population Health Survey, (1994, 1996, 1998). The sample is composed only of individuals whose mother tongue is not one of the Canadian official languages.	A measure of network intensity obtained as the product of a measure of contact availability (i.e., supply of residents in community *j* sharing the same mother tongue *k* of the individual) and a measure of average utilization of health care services by language group *k*.	(1) Having visited a general practitioner, (2) having visited a dentist, (3) having a regular doctor, and (4) having had a generic interaction with the health care system	Community and language group fixed effects, plus instrumental variables to account for individuals' self-selection in communities. Instruments are the measures of network and contact availability calculated on a more aggregated area.	Networks (peer effects) increase the probability of the first contact with the health care system.
Fiorillo and Sabatini, 2011	Italy, Multipurpose Survey on Household (Italian Institute of Statistics), round 2000	Frequency of meeting with friends	Self-reported health	Instrumental variables linear probability model (and other models) with regional fixed effects. Instruments are the individual propensity to talk about politics and the wealth of informal ties of the community where the individual lives.	Structural social capital improves the health conditions of individuals.

(*Continued*)

Table 7.1: (Continued)

Reference	Country/Dataset/ Year	Social Capital Indicators	Health Outcomes	Method	Results
Folland et al., 2007	US, 48 states over 1975–1998 at four-year intervals. Data are from DDB Life Style Database 1975–1998 generated by DDB Worldwide of Chicago	At the community level only. US state and time average of social capital index based on frequency of attendenace at club meetings, working for community projects, entertaining people at home, volunteer work, agreement on "most people are honest," time spent with friends.	Total mortality, infant mortality, proportion of people who are underweight, heart mortality, cancer mortality, accident mortality, suicide rate	Random effect panel analysis and instrumental variable estimates (without state fixed or random effects). Instruments are employment rate, latitude, state contributions to college education.	Social capital has the expected and significant sign in 3 out 7 health outcomes in the random effect model and 4 out 7 in the IV analysis. However, for health and infant mortality the effect goes in the opposite direction and is significant.
Fujiwara and Kawachi, 2008	US, National Survey of Midlife Development in the U.S. (MIDUS), 1995, 2007	At the individual level only: Social trust, sense of belonging, time devoted to volunteer work, participation in religious services and social organizations	Self-reported physical health, self-reported mental health, number of depressive symptoms, an index of major depression, based on the Composite International Diagnostic Interview Short Form (CIDI-SF)	Twins fixed effect (first difference between each pair of twins), distinguishing between monozygotic and dizygotic twins: the former share both genetic endowment and family background, while the latter share only the same family background.	In monozygotic twins, social trust positively and significantly influences self-reported physical health. No effect of other social capital measures on any of the health indicators. In dizygotic twins, the link between social capital and health is stronger (but the sample size is much larger). The difference between the coefficients of social trust on self-rated physical health among DZ and MZ is not significant, suggesting that effects of genetic factors on the association between social trust and self-rated physical health are small.

(Continued)

Table 7.1: (Continued)

Reference	Country/Dataset/ Year	Social Capital Indicators	Health Outcomes	Method	Results
Rocco *et al.*, 2011	25 European Countries, European Social Survey (ESS), 2002, 2004, 2006, 2008	At the individual level, generalized trust. At the community level, average generalized trust of each individual's reference group. Reference groups are defined according to individual age such that they partially overlap	Self-reported health	Two simultaneous equations with contemporaneous variables. One relates health to individual and community social capital, and one relates individual social capital to individual health and community social capital. Health, individual social capital and community social capital are treated as endogenous. They are categorical variables, and a simultaneous two-step ordered probit model is estimated. The identifying variables that are excluded are direct experience of a burglary and measures of health care supply in the first and second equation, respectively.	The causal relationship between social capital and health is circular. The effect of individual social capital to health largely exceeds that of community social capital. As a robustness check, misreporting in individual social capital is modeled and accounted for. Results are also confirmed in this case.

(Continued)

Table 7.1: (Continued)

Reference	Country/Dataset/ Year	Social Capital Indicators	Health Outcomes	Method	Results
Ronconi et al., 2010	Argentina, Encuesta de Desarrollo Social (EDS), 1997. The sample includes individuals aged 65+	Index of informal social interactions based on the frequency with which the respondent meets friends and relatives and whether the respondent lives alone.	Self-reported health	Instrumental variable model, with locality fixed effects (there are 113 localities). Instruments, which vary at the individual level, are: (1) whether there is public transportation in the neighborhood (binary variable) and (2) whether the person reports that transportation is an important problem in her/his life (binary variable). Distance from the nearest hospital and possibility of local contamination are controlled for. Analysis is conducted separately for men and women.	Significant effect of social capital on health for both men and women. Instruments (especially the second) are strong, and the over-identification test is largely passed.
Scheffler et al., 2007	US, National Health Interview Survey, 1999, 2000, 2001	Petris Index at the metropolitan statistical area (58 MSAs)	K6 index for non-specific psychological distress	Multi-Level (2 levels) analysis: Level 1, individual; level 2 MSA. Social capital variable is lagged one period. MSA dummies are included to capture unobserved area heterogeneity. Analysis done	Significant beneficial effect of social capital on mental health among individuals below median income when area dummies are included. Inclusion of MSA dummies

(Continued)

Table 7.1: (Continued)

Reference	Country/Dataset/ Year	Social Capital Indicators	Health Outcomes	Method	Results
				separately for above/below median family income.	altered level-two estimates significantly, suggesting that level-two random effects are correlated with included variables and so fail to meet multi-level analysis assumptions.
Sirven, 2006	Madagascar, rural area of Antsirabe, 587 households in 2001	Group participation, collective actions, giving or receiving remittances, organizing traditional ceremonies	Self-reported index based on the question "Would you say your needs in the domain of health are fulfilled?"	Two-step procedure. First, social capital indicators are regressed on household characteristics. Next, the predicted social capital and the residual are included in a second-stage equation whose outcome is health, excluding most of the first-stage predictors. Each social capital measure is considered separately. This is not to be interpreted as an IV analysis	Collective action and inclusion in a remittances network is positively associated with health.

(Continued)

Table 7.1: (Continued)

Reference	Country/Dataset/ Year	Social Capital Indicators	Health Outcomes	Method	Results
Sirven and Debrand, 2011	11 European countries, Survey on Health, Ageing, and Retirement in Europe (SHARE), Waves 1 (2004), 2 (2006), plus SHARELIFE (retrospective)	At the individual level only. Participation in social activities (voluntary/charity work, training courses, sports/social clubs, religious organizations, and political/community organizations)	(Poor) self-reported health, limitations in ADLs, limitations in usual activities, limitations in mobility, low grip strength, depressive symptoms (EURO-D scale), relative cognitive impairments (index derived from a cognitive score based on a memory test and a test of executive functions)	The sample is composed of individuals aged 50+. System of two dynamic equations that relate current health (resp. social capital) to lagged social capital and health. Individual unobserved heterogeneity is parameterized by means of retrospective information (initial conditions) and the time average of exogenous controls. The system is estimated by means of ML estimator (bi-variate probit).	Taking part in social activities at time t reduces respondents' probability of poor health at time $t + 1$ for all health indicators except grip strength. On the other hand, being in poor health at time t reduces the chances that an individual will take part in social activities at time $t + 1$ for all health measures. The impact of health on social capital is significantly higher than the social capital's effect on health.
Yamamura, 2010	Japan, Social Policy and Social Consciousness (SPSC) Survey 2000	Involvement in a neighborhood association	Self-reported health	Instrumental variable model. The instrument is a homeowner dummy.	Social capital has a significant positive effect on health status for unemployed people but not for employed people.

could provide, at best, an indication of an instrument's validity, but these tests are not conclusive, as they lack statistical power. Since the value of the test statistics declines when estimates are imprecise, a common occurrence with IV, such tests tend to under-reject the null of exogeneity (which is accepted when the test statistics approaches zero), so they tend to provide over-optimistic indications. On the other hand, if IV estimates are precise, a rejection would not necessarily imply that the instrument is bad; instead, it could point to a misspecification of the model's functional form or to a heterogeneous effect of social capital.

We find a wide set of instruments proposed in the literature. Brown *et al.* (2011) instrument CSC, measured by the Petris Index, with weather characteristics and ethnic heterogeneity at the county level and find that social capital significantly reduces smoking. d'Hombres *et al.* (2010) also use indices of community heterogeneity in terms of income, education, and religion and the average of CSC indicators as an instrument for ISC. Deri (2005) instruments CSC with a measure of social capital in a larger area. Folland (2007), by exploiting variation among states in the US, uses geographical latitude and state contributions to college education as instruments. Although all these instruments pass over-identification tests, and although there are good reasons behind their excludability, some concerns remain. They are all defined at the community level, so they could be correlated with relevant unobservable community characteristics. In cross-sectional data this problem cannot be addressed by including community dummies; otherwise, there would be perfect multi-collinearity with the instrument. In panel or pseudo-panel analysis, the small or null over time variation of instruments, such as community heterogeneity and latitude, could be insufficient to create a strong correlation with social capital when community and time dummies are included. In this case the requirement that the instruments be relevant could be at risk. In an attempt to increase instruments' variability in a cross-section regression with community fixed effects, d'Hombres *et al.* (2010) compute averages and heterogeneity indices over the set of residents in the community, excluding the respondent. This strategy introduces enough individual variation to prevent perfect multi-collinearity. Nevertheless, instruments' results are rather weak. A step forward has been made by Ronconi *et al.* (2010), who instrument ISC using variables defined at the individual level so community fixed effects can be safely included. However, in Ronconi *et al.* (2010) instruments are self-reported variables (whether there is lack of public transportation in the neighborhood and whether transportation is an important problem in the respondent's life), whose reporting could be influenced by unobservable individual characteristics. If so, the omission of individual characteristics would threaten the instrument's validity.[24]

Two papers, Sirven and Debrand (2011) and Rocco *et al.* (2013), recognize that social capital influences health and that people in better health could accumulate more social capital. Therefore, the relationship between the two variables is circular. Both papers make use of a cross-country dataset and define two-equation models. Sirven and Debrand (2011) exploit longitudinal information and relate current health with lagged social capital and social capital with health so the equations are not properly simultaneous; simultaneity derives instead from the assumed correlation between the error terms of the two equations. Individual heterogeneity is explicitly parameterized by exploiting retrospective information referring to individual childhood. The model is estimated by a maximum likelihood bi-variate probit estimator. Rocco *et al.* (2013), on the other hand, explicitly model the simultaneous circular relationship between social capital and health. As in standard simultaneous equation models, identification of the structural parameters is achieved by means of exclusion restrictions. (See Wooldridge, 2002, Chapter 9 for a comprehensive treatment of simultaneous equation models.) In particular, having being victim of a burglary or an assault is an explanatory variable included in the social capital equation but excluded from the health equation. Symmetrically, measures of health care supply are included in the health equations but are excluded from the social capital equation. The plausibility of the exclusion restrictions depends on a long battery of controls included in both equations.[25] As both social capital and health are categorical variables, a two-step ordered probit estimator is employed, as derived in Stern (1989). Both papers find that social capital and health are part of a circular relationship. Rocco *et al.* (2013) show that this result is robust to alternative definitions of community (reference groups) and to the possibility that individuals misreport social capital (generalized trust in the paper).

---

[24]Along the same lines, Yamamura (2011) uses a dummy indicating whether the individual is a homeowner or not, and Fiorillo and Sabatini (2011) instrument social capital with both the individual propensity to talk about politics and the wealth of informal ties at the aggregate level.

[25]Exclusion restrictions in a simultaneous equation model are essentially instrumental variables. An excluded variable serves as the instrument for one included endogenous variable. For this reason simultaneous equation models belong to the class of the IV estimators.

According to Sirven and Debrand (2011), who use an index of participation in social organizations as a measure of social capital and who focus on individuals over age 49, the feedback effect from health to social capital is stronger than the direct effect from social capital to health.

In order to control for individual family background, early health conditions, and genetic endowment, Fujiwara and Kawachi (2008) compare pairs of monozygotic (MZ) and dizygotic (DZ) twins. By first differencing social capital (measured by social trust), self-reported health, and other controls between twin pairs they remove common unobservables and make it possible to show that the association between social capital and health does not depend on common experiences in the twins' early lives or their common genetic endowment. Actually, the estimates obtained separately from the sample of MZ twins (common genetic endowment) and DZ twins (partially different genetic endowment) are not significantly different, suggesting that genetic endowment does not play a central role. However, as Diez Roux (2008) points out, twin fixed effects cannot control for the life-course and adult experiences, which are likely to differ. Moreover, the possibility of a spurious correlation between social capital and health because both variables are self-reported is not necessarily resolved by first differencing. The possibility of reverse causation also remains open. Nonetheless, the strategy of comparing twins is worth considering.

Associations

The large majority of all published papers in the field are papers that study the association between social capital and health. Although many countries have been studied, attention is mainly devoted to the US and the UK and other European countries. The majority of the studies look at a single country (or even one US state), although several papers report cross-country analysis. Among these, three are based on the European Social Survey, and one exploits the World Value Survey. More than 60 percent of the papers reviewed in this section adopt a multi-level strategy, where both ISC and CSC indicators are included at different levels. The remaining papers opt for alternative multivariate regression-based estimators (Table 7.2).

Multi-level analysis treats ISC and other individual characteristics as a level-one variables and CSC and other community factors as a level-two variables. The definition of community, which is often dictated by data availability, ranges from

Table 7.2: Selected recent studies that look for associations between social capital and health.

Reference	Country/Dataset/ Year	Social Capital Indicators	Health Outcomes	Method	Results
Baron-Epel *et al.*, 2008	Israel 2004–2005, distinguishing between Jews and Arabs	Social trust, neighborhood safety, perceived helpfulness, trust in local and national authorities, social support, social contacts	Self-reported health	Multivariate logistic regression separately for Jews and Arabs. Indicators interacted with an ethnicity dummy on the entire sample, including social capital. Controls included: sex, age, income, education, employment, marital status, and religiosity.	Jewish respondents with higher social capital reported better health. Among Arabs, only social support was significantly associated with health, although the sign of the other social capital measures was positive. The association is systematically weaker among Arabs than Jews, although the difference is not statistically different, except for social support.
Berry and Welsh, 2010	Australia, Household, Income and Labour Dynamics in Australia (HILDA) Survey, wave 6	Community participation: Frequency of individual types of participation, breadth across types of participation and perceptions about participation; index of informal social connectedness based on trust, reciprocity, social cohesion	Mental health was measured using the mental health subscale of the SF-36. Physical health was measured using two subscales of the SF-36: The transformed general health and physical functioning subscales. Scores for all three scales range from 0 to 100.	Correlation analysis and multi-level analysis for mental health, controlling for physical health. All social capital indicators are included simultaneously.	Social capital is related to better general physical and mental health, although the connection with the latter is stronger. The relationship between social capital and mental health is not due to physical health.

(Continued)

Table 7.2: (Continued)

Reference	Country/Dataset/ Year	Social Capital Indicators	Health Outcomes	Method	Results
Borgonovi, 2010	UK, cohort 1958 (NCDS) and cohort 1970 (BCS) over the lifecycle	Membership in groups or associations, religious attendance, generalized trust, voting in the last national election	Self-reported health, self-reported limiting and long-lasting illness, unhealthy behaviors (obesity and alcohol abuse), malaise, dissatisfaction	Probit model estimates that include only contemporaneous information are compared with the estimates produced by specifications that include the health and socio-economic conditions when the individual was child (lifecycle approach).	Observed associations between social capital and health indicators are robust to the inclusion of controls for childhood circumstances. The finding on the robustness of estimates of the association between social capital and health when adopting a lifecycle approach holds under different specifications are similar across birth cohorts, genders, and socio-economic groups.
Brown et al., 2006	US, NHIS 1998–2000	Petris Index and proportion of the Petrix Index that is due to religious association. Social capital is measured at the Metropolitan Statistical Area level	Smoking condition and number of cigarettes per day	Two-part model: A linear probability model estimates smoking condition and a generalized negative binomial model to estimate the number of cigarettes smoked. Metropolitan Statistical Area dummies are included in both. Controls are age, gender, race, income, education, price of cigarettes, and tobacco regulation indicators.	There is no effect of general community social capital. Instead, social capital related to religious organizations significantly reduces the number of cigarettes smoked although it has no significant effect on the individual smoking condition. This differential effect is suggested to be due to the strong nonsmoking norms in most religious groups.

(Continued)

Table 7.2: (Continued)

Reference	Country/Dataset/ Year	Social Capital Indicators	Health Outcomes	Method	Results
Fujisawa et al., 2009	Japan, original nationally representative survey, 2004	Individual social capital based on the following questions: "People in my neighborhood are willing to help if someone needs help" (perceived helpfulness), "People in my neighborhood are willing to take care of their neighbor's house while they are away" (kindness), and "People in my neighborhood usually exchange greetings" (greeting). Further, the responses to these items were combined to create the social cohesion index. At the community level, social capital is the average of individual social capital indicators.	General health perception index based on the common self-reported health and answers to "I seem to get sick a little easier than other people"; "I am as healthy as anybody I know"; "I expect my health to get worse"; "My health is excellent." All the items were combined to calculate the GH score, which ranged from 0 to 100.	Multi-level (2 levels) analysis: level 1 individuals; level 2 communities (i.e., clusters of about 50 households). One indicator of social capital is included in turn at both the individual and community levels.	Except kindness, all individual social capital indicators are significantly associated with health. Except perceived helpfulness, community social capital indicators are all (marginally) significant.
Giordano and Lindström, 2010	UK, BHPS, 1999–2005	Generalized trust; active participation in local community groups, local voluntary organizations, sport/leisure groups; use of informal networks; voting	Self-reported health	Separately for those in good and poor health in 1999, a logistic regression is performed to relate the change in health conditions to changes in explanatory variables between 1999 and 2005. All social capital indicators are included simultaneously.	Generalized trust and social participation are highly significantly associated with changes in self-rated health over time. Most other indicators of social capital are insignificant.

(Continued)

Table 7.2: (*Continued*)

Reference	Country/Dataset/ Year	Social Capital Indicators	Health Outcomes	Method	Results
Hurtado et al., 2011	Colombia, survey on a nationally representative sample of households in 27 of the 32 departments of Colombia and Bogotá, Capital District, 2004–2005	Generalized trust, reciprocity, membership (19 voluntary organizations), current voluntary activities, political participation, public civic activities.	Self-reported health	Multi-level (2 levels) analysis: level 1 Individual, level 2 department. All social capital indicators are included simultaneously (only at the individual level, as there is no significant variation in self-reported health at the department level).	Only generalized trust is significantly associated with health, after controlling for socio-demographic characteristics.
Hyyppa et al., 2007	Finland, Mini-Finland Health Survey, 1978–1980, followed up in 2004	Three social capital indices derived from factor analysis based on several indicators, including migration, residential stability, membership, friendship and trust.	Mortality (all causes and cardiovascular diseases)	Analysis conducted separately for males and females. Cox proportional hazard models, which relate the time of death to baseline social capital (1978–1980). Many specific health conditions and lifestyles are controlled for.	The social capital index related to trust is significantly associated with lower mortality for women and marginally significant for men. The other components of social capital are not associated with mortality.
Islam et al., 2006b	Sweden, Survey of Living Conditions (ULF survey), 1980/1981, 1988/1989, 1996/1997 — unbalanced individual panel	Average voting participation rate in municipal election, defined at the municipal level, over the period 1980–1997	Health status is measured by mapping responses to selected survey questions into the generic health-related quality of life measure EQ-5D	Multi-level (3 levels) linear model — level 1 is observations (one each time), level 2 is individual, and level 3 is municipality.	The small positive effect of social capital is significant only among males.

(*Continued*)

Table 7.2: (Continued)

Reference	Country/Dataset/ Year	Social Capital Indicators	Health Outcomes	Method	Results
Iversen, 2008	Norway, Standard of Living Survey and other sources, cross-section 1998 and panel 1997–2002	At the community level (county): proportion of people who attend church services, membership in sports organizations, voting turnout in local elections, fundraising per capita in national campaigns. At the individual level: the corresponding indicators.	Self-reported health; self-reported mental health	Multi-level analysis. In the cross-section case, 2 levels: individual and county. In the panel case, 3 levels: individual by time, individual, county. Social capital indicators are included simultaneously. Both individual and community indicators are included.	Voting turnout in local elections is positively associated with individual health in both cross-section and panel analysis. In the former model, voting turnout remains significant for general health only when individual voting is included.
Jusot *et al.*, 2008	France, Health, Health Care and Insurance Survey (ESPS), 2004	At the individual level only: membership in social organizations (also political.; trust, measured by the question, "Would you trust your neighbors to look after your children?"; social and emotional support.	Self-reported health	Separately for men and women. Logistic regression, where all social capital indicators are included simultaneously and where individual self-esteem, self-control, relative deprivation, and many socio-economic variables are controlled for.	Membership has a protective effect on health; trust is not associated with self-assessed health. Health status is positively associated with access to emotional support, rather than with the size of social networks.

(Continued)

Table 7.2: (Continued)

Reference	Country/Dataset/ Year	Social Capital Indicators	Health Outcomes	Method	Results
Kim and Kawachi, 2006	US, Social Capital Community Benchmark Survey, 2000 (40 communities, variously defined)	At the individual level, three indices of social capital derived from factor analysis (one pertaining to attitudes, one to social participation, and one to political participation). At the community level, weighted average of individual level indicators.	Self-reported health status	Multi-level (2 levels) model: level 1 individuals; level 2 communities. Both individual and community social capital are included simultaneously into the model. In one specification the interactions of the two are also included.	There is a modest (positive) association between each of three community social capital scales and self-rated health. Adding individual-level social capital variables to the model attenuates two of the three community social capital associations. Most individual-level social capital measures are strongly protective of health.
Kim et al., 2007	US, Behavioral Risk Factor Surveillance System (BRFSS) survey, 2001	At both the state and the county levels, a scale based on indicators that capture attitudes and social participation; a scale based on indicators that capture civic and political participation.	Obesity and physical activity during leisure time	Multi-level (2 levels) model: level 1 individuals, level 2, US states Multi-level (3 levels) model: level 1 individuals, level 2 counties, level 3 US states. Controls include Gini Index and income and racial composition.	There is a weak and usually not statistically significant association between social capital and both obesity and physical activity. Little support is found for social capital's mediating the associations of sprawl and income inequality with either outcome. There is some evidence of differential effects of social capital by race/ethnicity, particularly for American Indians/Alaska Natives (and Hispanics to a lesser extent) compared to Whites.

(Continued)

Table 7.2: (Continued)

Reference	Country/Dataset/ Year	Social Capital Indicators	Health Outcomes	Method	Results
Mansyur, 2008	45 countries, World Values Survey, 1990, 1995–1997	At the individual level: generalized trust, social participation (9 types of organizations). At the community level (country): average of trust and social participation.	Self-reported health	Muti-level (2 levels) analysis: level 1 individual; level 2 country. Control for individual income and Gini index. All indicators of social capital are included simultaneously at both levels.	Both social capital indicators at the individual level are positively associated with health. There is weak evidence of the role of community social capital and comparatively robust interaction effects between individual and community social capital.
Miller *et al.*, 2006	Indonesia, Indonesian Family Life Survey, 1993, 1997	Community-level social capital variable is the number of types of active community-level organizations (out of a possible 11). Communities (303) are defined as in IFLS.	Self-reported health, number of ADLs difficult to perform, fatigue, body pain	OLS regressions with the inclusion of individual and community characteristics. Standard errors are clustered at the community level.	Social capital is positively associated with good health across a variety of physical and mental health measures. There is mixed evidence for the existence of interactions between social capital and human capital.

(Continued)

Table 7.2: (*Continued*)

Reference	Country/Dataset/ Year	Social Capital Indicators	Health Outcomes	Method	Results
Nauenberg et al., 2011	Canada, Canadian Community Health Survey, 2002, Census 2001 and Ontario Health Ministry data 2006	Individual social capital is captured by attendance at religious services, social support, affection, marital status, living alone. Community social capital is measured by the Petris Index.	GP visits	Zero inflated negative binomial regression (non-utilization can be due to death between 2001 and 2006). Separately for census metropolitan areas (CMA) (pop >100,000) and census conglomeration areas (CA) (pop 10,000– 100,000).	Petris Index results are negatively associated with GP visits among CMA only. Individual social support results are negatively associated with GP visits in CMA, while religious attendance and affiliation in CA are positively associated with GP visits.
Olsen and Dahl, 2007	21 European countries, European Social Survey, 2002	Individual social capital is measured by the intensity of relationships with friends, relatives, and colleagues. Community social capital is measured by social trust.	Self-reported health	Multi-level (2 levels) analysis: level 1 individuals, level 2 countries.	Individual social capital is always significantly associated with health, similarly for men and women. Community social capital is unrelated to health.
Petrou and Kupek, 2008	England, Health Survey for England, 2003	Only individual social capital measures: trust/reciprocity, social support, civic participation.	Health-related quality of life (EQ-5D) and self-reported general health	Regression analysis	Low stocks of social capital across the domains of trust and reciprocity, perceived social support, and civic participation are significantly associated with poor measures of health status.

(*Continued*)

Table 7.2: (Continued)

Reference	Country/Dataset/ Year	Social Capital Indicators	Health Outcomes	Method	Results
Poortinga, 2006a	Europe (22 countries), European Social Survey, round 1, 2002	Social trust index (derived from three questions related to generalized trust) and social participation index (derived from participation in 12 kinds of social organizations). Community social capital is the average of individual social capital.	Self-reported health	Multi-level (2 levels) model: level 1 individuals; level 2 country. Individual and community social capital are included jointly.	Individual social capital is strongly associated with health, while there is no statistically significant association between community social capital and health, conditional to individual social capital. Moreover, the effect of individual social capital is larger when community social capital is higher. These results confirm Subramanian *et al.*'s (2002) results for the US.
Poortinga, 2006b	England, Health Survey for England, 2000, 2002	At the individual level: index of social support, generalized trust, participation in 14 voluntary organizations. At the community level: average of individual generalized trust and social participation and average of answers to the question "This area is a place where neighbors look after each other."	Self-reported health	Multi-level (3 levels) random coefficient model: level 1 individuals; level 2 household; level 3 sample point.	Individual social capital is positively associated with health. As for community social capital, only aggregate generalized trust remains statistically significant when individual social capital and other individual and contextual controls are included.

(Continued)

Table 7.2: (Continued)

Reference	Country/Dataset/ Year	Social Capital Indicators	Health Outcomes	Method	Results
Rostila, 2007	20 European countries, European Social Survey, 2002	At the individual level, generalized trust. Community social capital is trust averaged at the country level.	Self-reported health	Multi-level (2 levels): level 1 individuals; level 2 country. Indicators of the welfare-type regime adopted by each country are included and are also interacted with individual trust.	Individual trust is positively associated with health, but community social capital has no significant effect. There is significant heterogeneity of the effect of social capital across welfare regimes, which is especially low in countries that adopted the post-socialist regime.
Scheffler et al., 2008	US, Northern California member of the Kaiser Permanente integrated health care delivery system hospitalized for acute coronary syndrome between 1998 and 2002	Petris Index measured at the county level	Acute coronary syndrome	The purpose of the paper is to find an association between community-level social capital and the recurrence of acute coronary syndrome in the period 1998–2002 by making use of retrospective clinical data on the first occurrence. Multi-level (3 levels) Cox proportional hazard model: level 1 individual, level 2 census block-group, level 3 county.	Higher community social capital reduces the recurrence of acute coronary syndrome among those living in census block groups with lower than median income.

(Continued)

Table 7.2: (*Continued*)

Reference	Country/Dataset/ Year	Social Capital Indicators	Health Outcomes	Method	Results
Snelgove et al., 2009	UK, BHPS, 1998, 1999, 2003	At the individual level: Generalized trust, participation in voluntary organizations (16 different types of organizations). At the community level (i.e., postcode sector, the primary sampling unit of BHPS): average of generalized trust and civic participation.	Self-reported health	Multi-level (2 levels) analysis: level 1 individuals; level 2 postcode sectors. The outcome is self-reported health in 2008. Social capital variables refer to 2003. Baseline health in 2008 is included as control.	Both individual and community generalized trust are positively and significantly associated with health, while civic participation has no effect. There is no significant interaction between individual and community social capital.
Yip et al., 2007	China, baseline survey of a longitudinal study conducted in three rural counties of Shandong Province during March/April 2004	Membership in party organizations, membership in voluntary organizations, trust index (based on 12 questions related to trust, reciprocity, mutual help). Village-level social capital indicators are average levels of membership and trust at the village level.	Self-reported general health, psychological health, and subjective well-being	Multi-level (2 levels) analysis: level 1 individuals; level 2 villages (48); all indicators of social capital are included simultaneously at both levels.	Social capital is positively associated with general health, psychological health, and overall well-being. There is also evidence that social capital may operate independently at the individual and village levels. The trust index exhibits the most consistently positive associations with all three outcome indicators.

a municipality to a county, a state, and a country (in the cross-country studies). Which is the "correct" definition of community remains an open question in the literature. The community level one chooses may differ depending on the social capital indicator adopted and on which mechanisms that link social capital and health one wants to study. If the purpose of a study is to identify the role of informal social support, then defining communities as municipalities or neighborhoods seems more appropriate. If the Petris Index, a measure based on employment in non-profit organizations, is adopted as a measure of CSC, it seems reasonable to define the relevant community so it approximates the borders of the local labor market. The choice of the community should also take into account that, because of the smaller sample, measurement errors are typically larger when social capital indicators are computed over smaller communities. On the other hand, considering larger communities entails the risk of neglecting important geographical variability (modifiable area unit problem, Openshaw and Taylor, 1979).

Multi-level methods encompass a variety of methods to capture the hierarchical organization of data — that is, the fact that observations are nested. The most common example is that of individuals who are nested within communities (the two-level model). Panel data, where multiple observations per individual are available, can be used to estimate multilevel models in which level one is composed of individual-by-time observations of the same individual, individuals are level-two, and communities are level-three.[26] In the simplest multi-level models (the so-called random intercept model), the error term is composed of one component at each level. For instance, consider the health reduced-form model (7.1) and define $\varepsilon_{ij} = \mu_j + \phi_{ij}$, where a level-two random component μ_j is added to the level-one component ϕ_{ij}. More precisely μ_j is a level-two random shifter that assigns a specific intercept to each community. (The name "random intercept model" comes from here.) This structure introduces a correlation at level-two in the residuals ε_{ij} (clustering) that accounts for the hierarchical structure of the data.[27]

---

[26]See Islam *et al.* (2006b).

[27]More sophisticated variants of the model allow the introduction of random components, depending on some regressors. For instance, we could model $\varepsilon_{ij} = \mu_j + \theta_j SC_{ij} + \phi_{ij}$ so the random variable $\alpha + \theta_j$ becomes the resulting coefficient of SC_{ij}. This class of models is referred to as "random coefficient models."

Random intercept models are a generalization of the panel-data random effect model to the case in which there are n levels in the data hierarchy. In the simplest two-level case, multi-level models and panel data random-effect models are equivalent, and estimates are obtained by means of GLS. In order for GLS estimates to be unbiased and consistent, it must be assumed that μ_j is independent from all included regressors, whatever their level; that is, $E(\mu_j|Z) = 0$ for all $Z \in \{X_{ij}, W_j, SC_{ij}\}$. This assumption implies also that each regressor must be uncorrelated with the overall error term ε_{ij}; that is, each regressor, social capital included, must be exogenous. Therefore, random intercept models, as standard OLS, are not robust to endogeneity.

Blundell and Windmeijer (1997) show that, as the number of individuals per community tends to infinity, GLS estimates are consistent, even if μ_j is not independent from the included regressors. It follows that the appropriateness of multi-level models depends on the available data and the definition of community that has been adopted: The smaller the community, the smaller on average the number of observations available and the higher the risk of obtaining biased estimates. However, Blundell and Windmeijer's result holds only asymptotically, a situation rarely approached in practice by the available datasets.

Especially in studies that focus on social capital, the independence assumption on which multi-level models rely is unlikely to hold. Unobserved community-level characteristics related to local culture, history, and institutions are likely to be correlated with ISC and CSC and with the quality of the health care system and, ultimately, with individual health. Scheffler *et al.* (2007) check the plausibility of the independence assumption by introducing community-level fixed effect in a multi-level model and find that community-level estimates change significantly in both magnitude and sign. This result should encourage researchers to undertake multi-level model estimates with extreme care and to read their results as simple associations and, at best, as suggestive indications of the presence of a structural effect.

With this caution in mind, consider the results of the multi-level analyses we have reviewed, which generally find a strong association between social capital and health. Exceptions are Islam *et al.* (2006b), where a weak association between CSC and an index of quality of life emerges only among men, and Kim, Subramanian, Gortmaker and Kawachi (2006), where CSC indicators are weakly associated with obesity and physical activity. A significant association between health and ISC, CSC, or both emerges in all other studies. The inclusion of ISC often attenuates the effect of CSC. In Kim and Kawachi (2006), Olsen and Dahl (2007), and Poortinga (2006a), the association between CSC and health disappears when ISC is included; instead, ISC is always strongly associated with health.

Studies that do not adopt a multi-level approach generally confirm the finding of a strong association between ISC and health. Borgonovi (2010) exploits cohort studies and estimates the association between current health indicators and ISC by controlling for health and socio-economic conditions during childhood. Borgonovi finds that the association is not weakened by the inclusion of early-life controls. Somewhat in the same spirit, Hyppa *et al.* (2007) study whether ISC measured in the period 1978–1980 influences the time-to-death (with a cut-off at 2004). They find that social capital, when measured as an index based on trust, is associated with lower mortality, especially for women. Jusot *et al.* (2008) control for individual self-esteem, self-control, and relative deprivation in their logistic regressions and still find a significant association between self-reported health and membership in social organizations. However, they find no association between self-reported health and generalized trust, opening the possibility that common method bias is at work.

The inverse relationship: From health to social capital

A small body of literature examines the inverse effect, moving from health to social capital. Both Sirven and Debrand (2011) and Rocco *et al.* (2013) find a significant effect of health on social participation and trust. In their seminal paper, Alesina and La Ferrara (2002) find that the occurrence of traumas in the past year (such as diseases, accidents, divorce, or financial misfortune) is negatively associated with trust, although its effect tends to disappear quickly.

Shultz *et al.* (2009) estimate the association between the severe health conditions of a newborn and parents' participation in social organizations and religious attendance. The authors select children's exogenous health conditions (i.e., health conditions that are not the result of parents' behavior, such as Down syndrome and congenital heart malformations) that are associated with long-term consequences and find that infant health shocks do not reduce the social interactions of the child's parents. This finding confirms previous results obtained by Kazak and co-authors (1984, 1988).

Averett *et al.* (2010) test whether obese and overweight teen girls aged 14–19 are more likely to undertake risky sexual behaviors than girls who are of recommended weight. By means of a battery of alternative identification strategies that range from selection on observables to IVs and siblings' fixed effect, they find that overweight girls are less likely to be sexually active but that, when they are active, overweight girls are willing to take more risks than other girls are. The authors suggest that overweight girls compensate for their lower actual or perceived attractiveness with more willingness to incur greater risks in order to attract partners.

What do the measures of social capital really capture?

The study of the causal relationship between generalized trust and a number of economic and social variables is important in the social capital literature. The proxy for trust that researchers have used is usually the attitudinal measure of trust contained in surveys (e.g., the General Social Survey, or GSS). For example, the question "Generally speaking, would you say that most people can be trusted or that you can't be too careful in dealing with people?" (GSStrust) has been used as a measure of trust. Although the answers to such a question have been found to be statistically correlated to many factors, it is not completely clear which characteristic(s) the attitudinal trust question measures. Beginning with the seminal paper by Gleaser *et al.* (2000), many researchers have tried to disentangle the relationship between the attitudinal and the behavioral trust as measured both in experiments in the laboratory and in real life (e.g., the choice to lend). Glaeser *et al.*'s (2000) study takes into consideration the generalized trust (GSStrust) question and other two others from the same survey: "Do you think that most people try to take advantage of you if they got a chance?" (GSSfair) and "Would you say that most of the time people try to be helpful?" (GSShelpful). Glaeser *et al.* (2000) also consider a measure of past trusting behaviors.[28] To check the power of the questions in explaining trust, the answer to the attitudinal and behavioral questions in the surveys are related to the choices made in the contest of a *trust game* (also called *investment game*) played by Harvard students. In the trust game one player, the sender, receives an amount of money and decides how much to send to a second player, the recipient. The recipient has to decide how much he wants to send back to the sender. The game aims to measure both trust and trustworthiness.

---

[28]The subjects have to answer how often they lend personal possessions to friends, lend money to friends, and leave the door unlocked.

Glaeser *et al.* (2000) also consider the "envelope drop game," in which the experimenter tells the player that an envelope containing 10 dollars will be dropped in different places and in different situations and asks the player whether the envelope will be returned and with which amount of money. The results of the comparison between trust in surveys and trust in the lab show that attitudinal trust ascertained in the GSS survey predicts trustworthiness, not trust; the measure of past trust is better at predicting the trusting choices. In the last 10 years, the issue has been investigated by many authors with only minor changes in methodology. Ermish *et al.* (2009) modify the experimental design and confirm Glaeser *et al.*'s (2000) results using a subsample of the individuals interviewed in the British Household Panel Survey (BHPS). Fehr *et al.* (2003) replicate Glaeser *et al.*'s (2000) experiment using a sample of more than 400 German individuals from the German Socio-economic Panel Study (SOEP), finding results that are partially in contrast with Glaeser's results. In fact, both the attitudinal trust question (GSStrust) and the behavioral trust question performed well in predicting trusting behaviors in the lab, while none of the trust questions was a good predictor for trustworthiness. However, the questions lost their explanatory power once the authors controlled for expected transfers. Altruism seems to be another important factor in the determination of behaviors in the trust game: Capra *et al.* (2008) replicate Glaeser's results, but when they include altruism in the set of covariates, most of the trust questions (with the exception of GSStrust) have some explanatory power in predicting real actions.

Substantial independence between survey trust and trust measured in the trust game has been obtained using a sample of undergraduate students enrolled in the university of Liverpool (Vyrastekova and Garikipati, 2005), a sample of people studying in Linköping University in Sweden (Holm and Nystedt, 2008)[29] and a sample of 172 subjects in South Africa (Haile *et al.*, 2008).

Gachter *et al.* (2004) modify Glaeser's experimental set-up, substituting the trust game with a one-shot public good game with free-rider incentives, but the results are similar to those of the previous research: Neither the attitudinal nor the behavioral trust are correlated with the contribution to the public good, while GSSfair and GSShelp are. As in the Fehr *et al.* (2003) paper, the individual

---

[29]In this case, once the financial incentives are removed from the trust game, the correlation between the survey trust and the behavior in the laboratory becomes significant.

contribution is largely explained by beliefs about how much the others are willing to contribute to the common project.

Johansson-Stenman *et al.*[30] (2011) and Sapienza *et al.* (2007) find a strong correlation between the generalized trust question included in the world value survey and the behavior in the trust game. Sapienza *et al.* (2007) test the theory on a sample of approximately 500 students enrolled in the University of Chicago and detect a positive and significant correlation between the attitudinal generalized trust and the amount of money sent in a trust game. They also confirm that trustworthiness is correlated with the answer to the survey question (at least for high amounts of money sent). The explanation given for the partial difference between trust in survey and behavioral trust is that trust can be divided into two parts: A belief-related component and a preference-based one. While the behavior in the game captures both components, the question identifies just the belief-related component. Finally, Naef and Schupp (2009) find experimental trust to be correlated to a modified version of the GSS trust variable, the trust in strangers.[31]

Few papers have studied the links among trust measured in games, trust measured in the lab, and trust experienced in real situations. Karlan (2005) fills this gap considering around 800 individuals members of FINCA, a micro-credit program in Peru. The comparison between attitudinal trust and behavior in the trust game gives the usual response, that GSStrust predicts trustworthiness much better than trust, and Karlan finds the same pattern in comparing the lab setting with real-life choices. In fact, people who are classified as trustworthy in the game are those who are more likely to repay the loan, but those identified as trusting do not exhibit the same virtual behavior in the microcredit project and do not give the money back.

Monte Carlo Simulations

In this section we discuss the importance of the bias that is due to endogeneity when we estimate a health reduced-form model. As we cannot analyze all the

---

[30]In rural Bangladesh.

[31]The authors split the GSStrust and asked people whether they agree with four statements: (1) In general, you can trust people; (2) Nowadays, you can't rely on anybody; (3) How much do you trust strangers you meet for the first time; (4) When dealing with strangers, it is better to be cautious before trusting them.

possible sources of endogeneity, we focus on the case that plagues multilevel models: the presence of a correlation between the level-two component of the error term and ISC. This case of endogeneity can be generated when some community-level traits that are correlated with social capital and are relevant for individual health are omitted from the model. Scheffler *et al.* (2007) discuss this kind of problem, indicating as possible examples of omitted community traits "things as basic weather patterns, culture, local governmental policies, physical layout, and housing patterns" (p. 846).

The analysis is performed by means of a series of Monte Carlo experiments that allow us to analyze the behavior of an estimator in a controlled environment. The researcher artificially defines a data generating process (DGP) such that all relationships between the variables are perfectly known in advance. Next, the ability of an estimator to identify these relationships is tested by comparing estimates with the true parameters. The DGP we consider is simple: we suppose that individual health is the outcome of a linear function that includes only ISC, a community-level error component, and random noise. In line with the preceding discussion, we assume that ISC and the community-level error are positively correlated. Formally, the DGP is

$$h_{ij} = 1 + 0.15SC_{ij} + \mu_j + \phi_{ij} \qquad (7.8)$$

$$SC_{ij} = x_{1ij} + \mu_j \qquad (7.9)$$

where indices i and j refer, as usual, to individuals and communities, respectively; h_{ij} is individual health; SC_{ij} is ISC; and μ_j is the community effect. x_{1ij} is the exogenous component of ISC, which is uncorrelated with μ_j and ϕ_{ij}. Both x_{1ij} and μ_j are drawn from independent normal distributions, the former with mean 1 and standard deviation 2, the latter with mean 0 and standard deviation 2. The random noise, ϕ_{ij}, is normally distributed as well, with mean 0 and standard deviation 3. We chose these parameters in order to get roughly the same variation within and between communities in both social capital and health. By construction, the correlation between social capital and the community-level error is positive and strong (about 0.7). The causal (marginal) effect of social capital on health is fixed at 0.15.

We adopted six alternative estimators to estimate Eq. (7.10) with the data produced by our DGP.

$$h_{ij} = \alpha_0 + \alpha_1 SC_{ij} + \eta_{ij} \qquad (7.10)$$

The first one is the "naïve" OLS, which ignores the presence of unobservable community effects. The second and third are fixed (FE) and random (RE) effect estimators, respectively. Both recognize that the error term includes a community-level component, that is, that $\eta_{ij} = \mu_j + \phi_{ij}$, but the former allows for any correlation between SC_{ij} and μ_j, while the latter assumes no correlation. While, in general, the advantage of the former is that it is robust to any omission of community-relevant characteristics, the advantage of the latter is it produces efficient estimates (i.e., estimated standard errors are minimized), but at the cost of requiring much more exogeneity. Recall that the RE estimator is the same as the random intercept multi-level model.

Next we turn to IV procedures, distinguishing between two situations. In the first we dispose of an instrument generated within the DGP, Z_{ij}, which is correlated with x_{1ij} (correlation of 0.5) but uncorrelated with both community unobservables, μ_j, and the residual, ϕ_{ij}. In the second we dispose of a "less exogenous" instrument, ZZ_{ij}, defined as $ZZ_{ij} = Z_{ij} + \mu_j$, which is independent from ϕ_{ij} but positively correlated with μ_j. By adopting Z_{ij}, we ensure that the fourth estimator we look at is a pure IV. The last two estimators (the fifth and sixth) adopt the instrument ZZ_{ij} instead and include fixed (IVFE) and random (IVRE) community effects, respectively.

For each estimator we also consider six sample structures in terms of the number of communities and the number of residents in each community. In the first four structures the number of communities is fixed to 200, a number that is in line with those observed in the literature, while the number of individuals living in each community varies from 10 to 200. In the last two structures we keep the number of individuals per community constant at 100, and we increase the number of communities to 500 and 1,000, respectively. We look at alternative sample structures to study the asymptotic properties of the estimators along the community and individual dimensions and check Blundell and Windmeijer's (1997) result, which is that random effects converge to fixed effect estimates as the number of individuals per community goes to infinity.

Table 7.3 reports for each estimator and each sample structure the average point estimate of α_1, its standard deviation obtained from 500 replications, and the average of the standard errors analytically computed in each replication. If the estimator is unbiased, then the average point estimate will coincide with the true

Table 7.3: Monte Carlo simulations.

Sample Structure	Number of Communities	Number of Individuals	Ordinary Least Squares (OLS)	Fixed Effects (FE)	Random Effects (RE)	Instrumental Variables (IV)	Instrumental Variables with Fixed Effects (IVFE)	Instrumental Variables with Random Effects (IVRE)
1	200	10	0.650 (0.036) [0.026]	0.150 (0.035) [0.035]	0.576 (0.045) [0.028]	0.150 (0.081) [0.081]	0.148 (0.070) [0.071]	0.745 (0.052) [0.039]
2	200	50	0.647 (0.028) [0.012]	0.150 (0.015) [0.015]	0.561 (0.037) [0.013]	0.150 (0.036) [0.036]	0.150 (0.029) [0.030]	0.731 (0.039) [0.018]
3	200	100	0.647 (0.027) [0.008]	0.150 (0.011) [0.011]	0.561 (0.035) [0.009]	0.149 (0.025) [0.025]	0.149 (0.021) [0.021]	0.732 (0.036) [0.013]
4	200	200	0.647 (0.025) [0.006]	0.150 (0.007) [0.008]	0.559 (0.035) [0.006]	0.150 (0.019) [0.018]	0.150 (0.015) [0.015]	0.729 (0.035) [0.009]
5	500	100	0.650 (0.017) [0.005]	0.150 (0.006) [0.007]	0.560 (0.022) [0.006]	0.150 (0.016) [0.016]	0.150 (0.013) [0.013]	0.732 (0.023) [0.008]
6	1,000	100	0.649 (0.012) [0.004]	0.150 (0.005) [0.005]	0.560 (0.017) [0.004]	0.151 (0.011) [0.011]	0.151 (0.009) [0.010]	0.732 (0.017) [0.006]

Note: The average point estimate of social capital's effect on health (Eq. (7.10)), with over 500 replications. Standard deviations in parenthesis. Average analytical standard error in squared brackets.

marginal effect of the DGP (0.15 in our case). Moreover, the average analytical standard error should coincide with the standard deviation of the point estimate. We find that OLS estimates always suffer from a large upward bias since they do not take into account the strong positive correlation between social capital and community unobservables. Their analytical standard error is, conversely, systematically under-estimated. When community effects are included, the bias is reduced although random effect (RE) estimates are still largely upward-biased, given that the assumption of no correlation between SC_{ij} and μ_j is violated in our DGP. By contrast, fixed effect (FE) estimates are unbiased because they are robust to any correlation between SC_{ij} and μ_j. In this case analytical standard errors are also always correctly estimated.

Lack of bias is also achieved by the pure IV estimator. Although it will be difficult in practice to find instruments that are independent from μ_j, the IV procedure is effective in identifying the true marginal effect of social capital. Notice, however, that IV estimates are always less precise (i.e., they have a larger standard error) than FE estimates. Finally, with an instrument that is exogenous only conditional to the community effect (ZZ_{ij}), only IVFE estimates are unbiased, while IVRE are even more biased than simple RE and OLS.

In this analysis the extent of the bias in OLS and in random effect estimators is pronounced, as the estimates produced are four or five times larger than the true marginal effect. The bias is so large that it could even mask the true sign of the effect.[32] Even the dimension of the sample does not alter significantly the magnitude of the bias, although the asymptotic result obtained by Blundell and Windmeijer (1997) holds. The first four sample structures of Table A7.1 show the slow convergence of the RE estimates to the correct value as the size of the communities increases. Turning to the IV estimates, the use of endogenous IVs, as in the IVRE estimator, could generate biases even larger than those in OLS. The requirement of exogeneity is crucial in IV analysis.

However, these worrisome results depend on the degree of correlation between SC_{ij} and μ_j, which in our case is large for illustration purposes. With reference to the sixth sample structure (1,000 communities of 100 individuals each), if we

---

[32]This would have been the case if the true marginal effect had been zero or even moderately negative. Under this condition, the estimated effect obtained by OLS and the random effect models would have been positive anyway.

reduced the correlation from 0.70 to 0.45, the RE estimator bias would reduce by more than half (from 0.41, or 273 percent, to 0.17, or 112 percent). Further reducing the correlation to 0.10 reduces the RE bias to only 3 percent.[33] It is difficult to determine a plausible level for this correlation because it depends on multiple factors and is specific to the social capital indicator adopted. As an example, consider the last wave of the European Social Survey (collected in 2008 and covering many European countries). It includes 162 communities (defined as regions, according to NUTS 2 classification), with an average community size of 221 individuals, a situation close to our sample structure 4. The correlation among individual trust, the indicator of social capital considered, and community effects obtained by estimating Eq. (7.10) with a FE estimator is about 0.18. In this case the bias of RE would be about 10 percent.[34] Although moderate, such bias is not negligible.

Summary and Concluding Remarks

This chapter discusses the identification problems we encounter when we estimate the effect of social capital on health by means of a health reduced-form model and the empirical techniques adopted by the recent literature. We show that social capital must be treated as an endogenous variable in the empirical analysis and that the causes of endogeneity are: (1) Its two-way relationship with health, (2) its correlation with (probably) omitted variables, and (3) the measurement error that is likely to be embodied in the commonly used social capital indicators. We notice that the simultaneous inclusion of both ISC and CSC in the same equation could be problematic if CSC is computed as an average of ISC. Finally, we discuss the identification problems raised by Durlauf (2002) in the peer-effect settings, but we also suggest that adoption of the peer effect setting is less compelling if we are interested in the effect of the fundamental determinants of health on a given health outcome.

Looking at the literature published in the last five years, we argue that the multi-level analysis adopted by the majority of the papers, although appealing, rests on too-restrictive assumptions, which prevent the identification of causal effects. The

---

[33]It is 13 percent in sample structure 1 (the smallest sample size).
[34]It is likely that the inclusion of additional controls will further reduce such a correlation.

Monte Carlo experiment we conducted reveals that the size of the bias in the multi-level analysis estimates can be large and variable.

We also notice that the large majority of the recent studies adopt self-reported indicators of both social capital and health. The spurious correlation that is due to common methods bias could be important, but it has been largely overlooked.

The relatively few papers that explicitly look for causal effects usually adopt IV techniques. Certainly, the use of IV techniques goes in the right direction, and much progress has already been made, especially compared to earlier contributions, but there is still room for improvement. The conditions for instruments' validity — relevance and excludability — are sometimes debatable. The risk at stake is large, as non-excludable instruments could produce even larger biases than simple OLS does, regardless of their strength, as we see in the Monte Carlo experiment.

One potentially useful avenue to explore is that of exploiting historical shocks as exogenous sources of variation, as suggested by Becker *et al.* (2011) and Guiso *et al.* (2008b). Becker *et al.* (2011) consider the collapse of the Habsburg Empire and whether there is variation in terms of trust in the courts and police in the modern municipalities located on either side of the border of the former empire. Becker *et al.* and Guiso *et al.* find significant differences, indicating that history has long-term consequences for social capital. Guiso *et al.* (2008b) find similar results in comparing the Italian towns in northern Italy that were free city-states ("communes") in the 12th century with those that were not: The former today have higher levels of social capital than the latter, measured by the number of non-profit organizations, the presence of an organ donation association, and referenda turnout.

Besides producing firmer conclusions about the total effect of social capital on health, future research should endeavor effort to unveil the relative strength of the alternative mechanisms that channel the effect of social capital. We mentioned at the beginning of the chapter that social capital can operate with stronger social support, a more intense information flow, an enhanced lobbying capacity at the community level, and so on, but we know little about the importance of these channels, whether other mechanisms exist, and which ones should be targeted to make social capital an alternative tool for health policy. This agenda is long and compelling enough to keep researchers busy for awhile.

Appendix

Table A7.1: Principal datasets containing information on social capital and health

Dataset	Years	Type	Countries	Health Variables	Social Capital Variables	Sample Size	Access
The National Longitudinal Study of Adolescent Health (Add Health)	Longitudinal study of a nationally representative sample of adolescents in grades 7–12 in the 1994–1995 school year. Most recent wave: 2008.	Panel	USA	General health, disability, illnesses, mental health, BMI, smoking	Religion, friends and social networks, social activities	The number of Wave I respondents in this dataset is approximately 6,500 (public data).	Mainly public use after registration
British Household Panel Survey (BHPS)/ understanding society	18 waves, beginning in 1991 (annual)	Panel	UK	General health, longstanding illnesses and disability, smoking	Social support, political and social involvement, religion, social participation	Nationally representative sample of about 5,500 people in 1991 and about 10,000 interviewed individuals. Extension samples of 1,500 households in each of Scotland and Wales in 1999. In 2001 a sample of 2,000 households was added in Northern Ireland. Since 2009 the new British longitudinal survey has been called "understanding society," and the sample size has been around 40,000 households.	Free access after registration

Table A7.1: (Continued)

Dataset	Years	Type	Countries	Health Variables	Social Capital Variables	Sample Size	Access
English Longitudinal Survey of Aging (ELSA)	Annually from 2002/2003	Longitudinal	England	Generalized health, disability, longstanding illnesses, smoking, drinking, physical activity, mental health	Social support, social activities	Around 12,000 respondents from three separate years of the HSE survey were recruited to provide a representative sample of the English population aged 50 and over	Free access after registration
European Social Survey (ESS)	Round 1 (2002), round 2 (2004), round 3 (2006), round 4 (2008)	Repeated cross sections	All persons aged 15 and over resident within private households in more than 30 countries	General health, longstanding illnesses and disabilities	The themes covered in the core module are generalised trust, trust in institutions, political and social engagement, religion, socio-political values, moral and social values, social capital, social exclusion, and national, ethnic, and religious identity	Around 1,500–2,000 observations per country per wave	Free access after registration

(Continued)

Table A7.1: (Continued)

Dataset	Years	Type	Countries	Health Variables	Social Capital Variables	Sample Size	Access
European Values Survey (EVS)/ World values survey (WVS)	1981–1984, 1989–1993, 1994–1999, 1999–2004, 2005–2006	Repeated cross sections	World (87 countries)	General health,	Generalized trust, trust in specific groups and institutions, political and social engagement, religion, moral and social values	More than 256,000 interviews	Free access after registration
General Social Survey (GSS)	1972–2010	Repeated cross sections. panel since 2006	USA	General health	Generalized trust, religion	GSS has 5,415 variables, time-trends for 1,988 variables, and 257 trends having 20+ data points	Free
Health and Retirement Survey (HRS)	1992–2010, 12 waves (annually from 1992 to 1996, then every 2 years)	Panel	USA	Mental health, disability, longstanding illnesses, smoking, drinking, physical activity, BMI	Social capital variables that began in 2004 are social participation, friends	Surveys more than 22,000 Americans over the age of 50 every two years	Free access after registration

(Continued)

Table A7.1: (Continued)

Dataset	Years	Type	Countries	Health Variables	Social Capital Variables	Sample Size	Access
Health Survey for England, (HSE)	Contents 1992–2009	Repeated cross sections	England	General health, longstanding illnesses and disabilities, accidents, physical activity, eating habits, smoking, drinking	The first wave that contains social capital variables was collected in 2000. It contains information on social participation, friends, trust	12,413 (obtained) productive individuals in the 2000 wave	Free access via data archive
Multipurpose Survey on Households	From 1993 to 2003 the survey was conducted annually, with data collected during November. In 2004 the survey did not take place and, starting in 2005, it was run every year in February	Repeated cross sections	Italy	General health, nutrition, smoking, BMI	Social and political activities, religion, friends	Around 24,000	Restricted
National Child Development Study (NCDS)	8 waves between 1965 and 2009 (cohort study)	Longitudinal	UK	Generalized health, disability, smoking, drinking, accidents, mental health, diet, physical activity	The first wave that contains social capital variables is the fifth wave: social participation, generalized trust, politics, religion	Around 15,000 people in each wave	Free access after registration

(Continued)

Table A7.1: (Continued)

Dataset	Years	Type	Countries	Health Variables	Social Capital Variables	Sample Size	Access
National Health Interview Survey (NHIS)	From 1963, but part of the questionnaire changed beginning in 1997	Cross-sections	USA	Longstanding illnesses and disability, smoking	No social capital variables	Statistically representative sample of the US civilian non-institutionalized population. 35,000–40,000 households and about 75,000–100,000 individuals.	Free access
Panel Study of Income Dynamics (PSID)	36 waves from 1968 to 2009 (annually between 1968 to 1997, then biennially)	Panel	USA	Second wave: health limitations	Social and political activities, religion, social support	The PSID began in 1968 with a nationally representative sample of more than 18,000 individuals living in 5,000 families in the United States.	Mainly public use after registration
Survey of Health, Ageing and Retirement in Europe (SHARE)	3 waves: 1st wave (2004); 2nd wave (2006); 3rd wave Retrospective, Sharelife –retrospective data-(2008)	Panel	Over 50+ (and their spouses) from more than 20 countries in Europe	General health, longstanding illnesses, disabilities, BMI, smoking, physical activity, mental health	Social support, social and political activities	Around 30,000 for the first 2 waves and around 20,000 for the retrospective one	Free access after registration

References

Acemoglu, D. and Angrist, J. 2001. How large are human-capital externalities? Evidence from compulsory-schooling laws. In *NBER Macroeconomics Annual 2000, Volume 15*, eds. Bernanke, B.S. and Rogoff, K. Cambridge, Massachusetts: MIT Press.

Alesina, A. and La Ferrara, E. 2002. Who trusts others? *Journal of Public Economics*, 85(2): 207–234.

Angrist, J. D. and Pischke, J. S. 2008. *Mostly Harmless Econometrics: An Empiricist's Companion*. New Jersey: Princeton University Press.

Averett, S., Corman, H. and Reichman, N. 2010. Effects of overweight on risky sexual behavior of adolescent girls. National Bureau of Economic Research Working Papers, Vol. 16172.

Baron-Epel, O., Weinstein, R., Haviv-Mesika, A., Garty-Sandalon, N. and Green, M.S. 2008. Individual-level analysis of social capital and health: A comparison of Arab and Jewish Israelis. *Social Science and Medicine*, 66(4): 900–910.

Becker, S. O., Boeckh, K., Hainz, C. and Woessmann, L. 2011. The empire is dead, long live the empire! Long-run persistence of trust and corruption in the bureaucracy. CESifo Working Paper Series, Vol. 3392.

Berry, H. L. and Welsh, J. A. 2010. Social capital and health in Australia: An overview from the household, income and labour dynamics in Australia survey. *Social Science and Medicine (1982)*, 70(4): 588–596.

Bisin, A. and Verdier, T. 2010. The economics of cultural transmission and socialization. National Bureau of Economic Research Working Papers, Vol. 16512.

Blundell, R. and Windmeijer, F. 1997. Cluster effects and simultaneity in multilevel models. *Health Economics*, 6(4): 439–443.

Borgonovi, F. 2010. A lifecycle approach to the analysis of the relationship between social capital and health in Britain. *Social Science and Medicine*, 71(11): 1927–1934.

Brock, W. A. and Durlauf, S. N. 2001. Discrete choice with social interactions. *The Review of Economic Studies*, 68(2): 235–260.

Brown, T. T., Colla, C. H. and Scheffler, R.M. 2011. Does community-level social capital affect smoking behavior? An instrumental variables approach. Working paper presented at the 3rd Workshop of the Global Network on Social Capital and Health (Oslo, September 2010).

Brown, T. T., Scheffler, R. M., Seo, S. and Reed, M. 2006. The empirical relationship between community social capital and the demand for cigarettes. *Health Economics*, 15(11): 1159–1172.

Capra, C. M., Lanier, K. and Meer, S. 2008, Attitudinal and behavioral measures of trust: A new comparison. Available at http://ssrn.com/abstract=1091539.

Cooper, H., Arber, S. and Fee, L. 1999. The influence of social support and social capital on health: A review and analysis of British data. Health Education Authority, London.

De Giorgi, G., Pellizzari, M. and Redaelli, S. 2010. Identification of social interactions through partially overlapping peer groups. *American Economic Journal: Applied Economics*, 2(2): 241–275.

Deri, C. 2005. Social networks and health service utilization. *Journal of Health Economics*, 24(6): 1076–1107.

d'Hombres, B., Rocco, L., Suhrcke, M. and McKee, M. 2010. Does social capital determine health? Evidence from eight transition countries. *Health Economics*, 19(1): 56–74.

Diez Roux, A.V. 2008. The effects of social capital on health. What twin studies can tell us. *American Journal of Preventive Medicine*, 35(2): 182–183.

Durlauf, S. N. 2002. On the empirics of social capital. *The Economic Journal*, 112(483): F459–F479.

Durlauf, S. N. and Fafchamps, M. 2005. Social capital. In *Handbook of Economic Growth*, eds. Aghion, P. and Durlauf, S.N. pp. 1639–1699. Netherlands: Elsevier.

Ermisch, J., Gambetta, D., Laurie, H., Siedler, T. and Uhrig, N. 2009. Measuring people's trust. *Journal of the Royal Statistical Society: Series A (Statistics in Society)*, 172(4): 749–769.

Fehr, E., Fischbacher, U., von Rosenbladt, B., Schupp, J. and Wagner, G. 2003. A nation-wide laboratory: Examining trust and trustworthiness by integrating behavioral experiments into representative surveys. IZA Discussion Papers, number 715.

Fiorillo, D. and Sabatini, F. 2011. Quality and quantity: The role of social interactions in individual health. University of York Health, Econometrics and Data Group Working Paper, Vol. 11, No. 04.

Folland, S. 2007. Does 'community social capital' contribute to population health? *Social Science and Medicine*, 64(11): 2342–2354.

Fujisawa, Y., Hamano, T. and Takegawa, S. 2009. Social capital and perceived health in Japan: An ecological and multilevel analysis. *Social Science and Medicine*, 69(4): 500–505.

Fujiwara, T. and Kawachi, I. 2008. Social capital and health: A study of adult twins in the US. *American Journal of Preventive Medicine*, 35(2): 139–144.

Gachter, S., Herrmann, B. and Thoni, C. 2004. Trust, voluntary cooperation, and socio-economic background: Survey and experimental evidence. *Journal of Economic Behavior and Organization*, 55: 505–531.

Giordano, G. N. and Lindstrom, M. 2010. The impact of changes in different aspects of social capital and material conditions on self-rated health over time: A longitudinal cohort study. *Social Science and Medicine*, 70(5): 700–710.

Glaeser, E., Laibson, D., Scheinkman, J. and Soutter, C. 2000. Measuring trust. *Quarterly Journal of Economics*, 115(3): 811–846.

Grossman, M. 1972. On the concept of health capital and the demand for health. *The Journal of Political Economy*, 80(2): 223–255.

Guiso, L., Sapienza, P. and Zingales, L. 2008a. Alfred Marshall lecture: Social capital as good culture. *Journal of the European Economic Association*, 6(2–3): 295–320.

Guiso, L., Sapienza, P. and Zingales, L. 2008b. Long term persistence. National Bureau of Economic Research Work Papers, Vol. 14278.

Haile, D, Sadrieh, A. and Verbon, H. 2008. Cross-racial envy and underinvestment in South African partnerships. *Cambridge Journal of Economics*, 32(5): 703–724.

Holm, H. and Nystedt, P. 2008. Trust in surveys and games: A methodological contribution on the influence of money and location. *Journal of Economic Psychology*, 29(4): 522–542.

Hurtado, D., Kawachi, I. and Sudarsky, J. 2011. Social capital and self-rated health in Colombia: The good, the bad and the ugly. *Social Science and Medicine*, 72(4): 584–590.

Hyyppa, M. T., Maki, J., Impivaara, O. and Aromaa, A. 2007. Individual-level measures of social capital as predictors of all-cause and cardiovascular mortality: A population-based 22(9): 589–597.

Islam, M. K., Merlo, J., Kawachi, I., Lindström, M., Burstrom, K. and Gerdtham, U. G. 2006a. Does it really matter where you live? A panel data multilevel analysis of Swedish municipality-level social capital on individual health-related quality of life. *Health Economics, Policy, and Law*, 1(3): 209–235.

Islam, M. K., Merlo, J., Kawachi, I., Lindström, M. and Gerdtham, U. G. 2006b. Social capital and health: Does egalitarianism matter? A literature review. *International Journal for Equity in Health*, 5:3.

Iversen, T. 2008. An exploratory study of associations between social capital and self-assessed health in Norway. *Health Economics, Policy, and Law*, 3(4): 349–364.

Johansson-Stenman O., Mahmud M. and Martinsson P. 2011. Trust, trust games and stated trust: Evidence from rural Bangladesh. *Journal of Economic Behavior and Organization*, forthcoming.

Jusot, F., Grignon, M. and Dourgnon, P. 2008. Access to psycho-social resources and health: Exploratory findings from a survey of the French population. *Health Economics, Policy, and Law*, 3(4): 365–391.

Karlan, D. 2005. Using experimental economics to measure social capital and predict financial decisions. *American Economic Review*, 95(5): 1688–1699.

Kawachi, I., Kennedy, B. P., Lochner, K. and Prothrow-Stith, D. 1997. Social capital, income inequality, and mortality. *American Journal of Public Health*, 87(9): 1491–1498.

Kazak, A. E. and Marvin, R. S. 1984. Differences, difficulties and adaptation: Stress and social networks in families with a handicapped child. *Family Relations*, 33(1): 67–77.

Kazak, A. E., Reber, M. and Carter, A. 1988. Structural and qualitative aspects of social networks in families with young chronically ill children, *Journal of Pediatric Psychology*, 13(2): 171–182.

Kazak, A. E. and Wilcox, B. L. 1984. The structure and function of social support networks in families with handicapped children. *American Journal of Community Psychology*, 12(6): 645–661.

Kim, D. and Kawachi, I. 2006. A multilevel analysis of key forms of community- and individual-level social capital as predictors of self-rated health in the United States. *Journal of Urban Health: Bulletin of the New York Academy of Medicine*, 83(5): 813–826.

Kim, D., Subramanian, S. V., Gortmaker, S. L. and Kawachi, I. 2006. US state- and county-level social capital in relation to obesity and physical inactivity: A multilevel, multivariable analysis. *Social Science and Medicine*, 63(4): 1045–1059.

Laporte, A., Nauenberg, E. and Shen, L. 2008. Aging, social capital, and health care utilization in Canada. *Health Economics, Policy and Law*, 3(4): 393–411.

Lochner, K., Kawachi, I. and Kennedy, B. P. 1999. Social capital: A guide to its measurement. *Health and Place*, 5(4): 259–270.

Lindeboom, M., and van Doorslaer, E. 2004. Cut-point shift and index shift in self-reported health. *Journal of Health Economics*, 23: 1083–1099.

Lindström, M. 2007. Social capital and health-related behaviors. In *Social Capital and Health: A Decade of Progress and Beyond*, eds. Kawachi, I., Subramanian, S. V. and Kim, D., Springer.

Macinko, J. and Starfield, B. 2001. The utility of social capital in research on health determinants. *The Milbank Quarterly*, 79(3): 387–427.

Manski, C. F. 1993. Identification of endogenous social effects: The reflection problem. *The Review of Economic Studies*, 60(3): 531–542.

Mansyur, C., Amick, B. C., Harrist, R. B. and Franzini, L. 2008. Social capital, income inequality, and self-rated health in 45 countries. *Social Science and Medicine*, 66(1): 43–56.

Miller, D. L., Scheffler, R., Lam, S., Rosenberg, R. and Rupp, A. 2006. Social capital and health in Indonesia. *World Development*, 34(6): 1084–1098.

Muntaner, C., Lynch, J. and Smith, G. D. 2001. Social capital, disorganized communities, and the third way: Understanding the retreat from structural inequalities in epidemiology and public health. *International Journal of Health Services*, 31(2): 213–238.

Murgai, R., Winters, P., Sadoulet, E. and Janvry, A. 2002. Localized and incomplete mutual insurance. *Journal of Development Economics*, 67(2): 245–274.

Naef M. and Schupp J. 2009. Measuring trust: Experiments and surveys in contrast and combination. SOEP Paper No. 167.

Nauenberg, E., Laporte, A. and Shen, L. 2011. Social capital, community size and utilization of health services: A lagged analysis. *Health Policy*, 103(1): 38–46.

Olsen, K. M. and Dahl, S. 2007. Health differences between European countries. *Social Science and Medicine*, 64(8): 1665–1678.

Openshaw, S. and Taylor, P. 1984. *The Modifiable Areal Unit Problem*, Norwick: Geo Books.

Openshaw, S. and Taylor, P. J. 1979. A million or so correlation coefficients: Three experiments on the modifiable areal unit problem. In *Statistical Methods in the Spatial Sciences*, ed. N. Wrigley, London: Pion, pp. 127–144.

Petrou, S. and Kupek, E. 2008. Social capital and its relationship with measures of health status: Evidence from the Health Survey for England 2003. *Health Economics*, 17(1): 127–143.

Poortinga, W. 2006a. Social capital: An individual or collective resource for health? *Social Science and Medicine*, 62(1): 292–302.

Poortinga, W. 2006b. Social relations or social capital? Individual and community health effects of bonding social capital. *Social Science and Medicine*, 63(1): 255–270.

Rocco, L., Fumagalli, E. and Suhrcke, M. 2011. From social capital to health — and back. *Health Economics* (forthcoming).

Ronconi, L., Brown, T. T. and Scheffler, R. M. 2010. Social capital and self-rated health in Argentina. *Health Economics*, 21(2): 201–208.

Rostila, M. 2007. Social capital and health in European welfare regimes: A multilevel approach. *Journal of European Social Policy*, 17(3): 223.

Sapienza P., Toldra A. and Zingales L., 2007. Understanding trust. National Bureau of Economic Research. Working Papers, No. 13387.

Scheffler, R. M. and Brown, T. T. 2008. Social capital, economics, and health: New evidence. *Health Economics, Policy, and Law*, 3(4): 321–331.

Scheffler, R. M., Brown, T. T. and Rice, J. K. 2007. The role of social capital in reducing non-specific psychological distress: The importance of controlling for omitted variable bias. *Social Science and Medicine*, 65(4): 842–854.

Scheffler, R. M., Brown, T. T., Syme, L., Kawachi, I., Tolstykh, I. and Iribarren, C. 2008. Community-level social capital and recurrence of acute coronary syndrome. *Social Science and Medicine*, 66(7): 1603–1613.

Schultz, J., Corman, H., Noonan, K. and Reichman, N. E. 2009. Effects of child health on parents' social capital. *Social Science and Medicine*, 69(1): 76–84.

Sirven, N. and Debrand, T. 2011. Social capital and health of older Europeans. From Reverse Causality to Health Inequalities. IRDES Working Papers, No. 40.

Sirven, N. 2006. Endogenous social capital and self-rated health: Cross-sectional data from rural areas of Madagascar. *Social Science and Medicine*, 63(6): 1489–1502.

Snelgrove, J. W., Pikhart, H. and Stafford, M. 2009. A multilevel analysis of social capital and self-rated health: Evidence from the British Household Panel Survey. *Social Science and Medicine*, 68(11): 1993–2001.

Stern, S. 1989. Measuring the effect of disability on labor force participation. *Journal of Human Resources*, 24(3): 361–395.

Tabellini, G. 2010. Culture and institutions: Economic development in the regions of Europe. *Journal of the European Economic Association*, 8(4): 677–716.

Vyrastekova J. and Garikipati S. 2005. Beliefs and trust: An experiment. University of Liverpool Management School series of Research Papers, No. 200511.

Wilkinson, R. G. 1996. *Unhealthy Societies: The Afflictions of Inequality*, London: Psychology Press.

Wooldridge, J. M. 2002, *Econometric Analysis of Cross section and Panel Data*, Cambridge, Massachusetts: MIT Press.

Yamamura, E. 2010. Differences in the effect of social capital on health status between workers and non-workers. MPRA Paper, No. 22967.

Yip, W., Subramanian, S. V., Mitchell, A. D., Lee, D. T., Wang, J. and Kawachi, I. 2007. Does social capital enhance health and well-being? Evidence from rural China. *Social Science and Medicine*, 64(1): 35–49.

Chapter 8

Social Capital and Health in Low- and Middle-Income Countries

---

José Anchorena, Lucas Ronconi and Sachiko Ozawa

This chapter has three objectives. First, we set a series of questions related to the trio of social capital, health, and economic development to determine whether the positive correlation between social capital and health that has been observed in high-income countries also holds in low- and middle-income countries. We also address whether different forms of social capital (e.g., informal interactions, participation in organizations, trust) have different effects on health, depending on the level of economic development and whether the mechanisms driving the correlation between social capital and health differ in richer and poorer countries. Second, we review the econometric literature of social capital and health in developing countries. The evidence suggests that social capital is positively correlated with health in developing countries, but coefficients are not strictly comparable with those for developed countries because of differences in data, measures, and methodologies. Third, we compute and compare the correlations for a number of developing and developed countries using a homogenous international dataset (i.e., the International Social Survey Programme, or ISSP), which, to our knowledge, has not been used for this type of study before. We also use a local household survey to present results for more and less developed regions of Argentina, a country in which there is significant heterogeneity of income across provinces. Overall, we find that correlations between participation in organizations and health are usually of similar magnitude across richer and poorer countries (or regions), but trust has a larger positive association with health in more developed countries. We conclude by pointing out directions for further research.

Conceptual Framework: Forms of Social Capital and Types of Health Problems

How does the relationship between social capital and health evolve with economic development? The answer to this question is determined by how we define social capital and health.

There is much discussion about the definition of social capital, with the main divide being between those who define social capital as *an attribute of persons* and those that define social capital as *connections between persons*.[35] The first group considers the *degree of trust* as a good measure of social capital (e.g., Guiso *et al.*, 2004), while the second group considers the *number, intensity, and structure of social ties* as measures of social capital (e.g., Coleman, 1988). Of course, both concepts (attributes and connections) may be related, although surprisingly little work has been done in that respect: A high degree of trust may increase the number and intensity of certain types of social ties, and a high number of social ties and/or the intensity of these ties may increase the degree of trust.

Moreover, within the camp that sees social capital as a network of connections, different researchers emphasize different types of ties. There are three main types of ties: family ties, friends' ties, and civic associations' ties (also called secondary organizations' ties, such as political parties, religious meetings, clubs, and unions). Across countries, there is evidence that the number and intensity of family ties are negatively associated with economic development, while the number of friends' and secondary organizations' ties are positively associated with development (Table 8.1). Development has been found to be negatively associated with the intensity of friends' ties, which are measured by the frequency of visits (Anchorena and Anjos, 2008).

There is less controversy about the definition of health, but there are different burdens of disease, and the relationship between social capital and health will depend on the diseases to which we refer. For our purposes, the main classification we discuss is that between physical and mental health, but it is also important to

---

[35] Moreover, Solow (2000) and Arrow (2000) have expressed doubt in the usefulness of the concept, and some of those doubts remain, despite the wealth of studies and the progress made. Solow (2000) says that social capital does not imply an essential characteristic of "capital," a "deliberate sacrifice in the present for future benefit," while Arrow (2000) asks, "What is social capital a stock of?" and suggests calling it "patterns of behavior" instead.

Table 8.1: Correlations among network social capital indicators, income per capita, and incidence of neuropsychiatric diseases.

Variable		GDP pc	Incidence Neuro/Total
Nuclear Family	Number	**−0.51**	−0.32
		0.007	0.11
	Intensity	**−0.58**	**−0.45**
		0.002	0.02
Friends	Number	**0.54**	**0.41**
		0.004	0.04
	Intensity	**−0.67**	**−0.63**
		0.002	0.0005
Secondary Associations	Number	**0.64**	0.34
		0.0005	0.09
	Intensity	0.054	0.27
		0.79	0.18

Note: Correlations are computed over the means of 26 countries. "GDP pc" denotes per capita gross domestic product, while "incidence neuro/total" refers to the ratio of the number of age-standardized disability-adjusted years of life lost because of neuropsychiatric diseases to those that are lost because of all types of diseases. "Number" refers to the number of ties (e.g., number of members in the nuclear family), while "intensity" refers to the intensity of the ties (as measured by frequency of visits). Below the correlation coefficient we indicate the p-value associated with it. Correlations significant at the 5% level are in bold.

Source: For measures of social capital, Anchorena and Anjos (2008), based on ISSP (International Social Survey Programme); for the health measure, World Health Organization (see below).

distinguish between the types of physical health problems, that is, communicable diseases, non-communicable diseases, and injuries.

The evidence indicates a strong positive association between indicators of physical health and income per capita (see Figure 8.1). According to data from the World Health Organization, an average high-income country (i.e., more than US$20,000 PPP in 2004) has 31 percent of the age-standardized disability-adjusted life years (DALYs, which we want to avoid) per 100,000 of those in a low-income country (i.e., less than US$5,000 PPP in 2004). The ratio is only 5 percent for communicable diseases, 53 percent for non-communicable diseases, and 33 percent for injuries, but it is 103 percent for neuropsychiatric causes (Table 8.2). This finding denotes the different burden of disease faced by countries in different

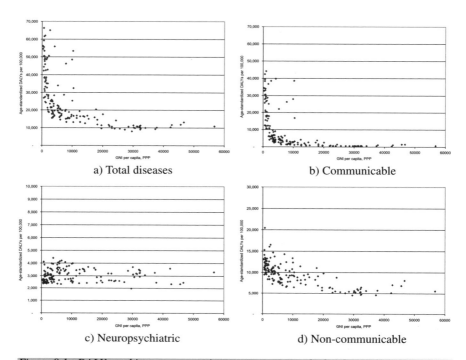

Figure 8.1: DALYs and income per capita across countries, by burden of disease.
Note: Each dot is a country. Income per capita is measured in USD.
Source: See Table 8.2.

stages of economic development. Many low- and middle-income countries face a double burden of disease, with a high prevalence of both communicable and non-communicable diseases. When one distinguishes these different types of social capital and burden of disease, one may find a complex picture of the development of the relationship between social capital and health.

Mechanisms: Personal and institutional factors

The patterns of interaction between economic development and different types of social capital and health point to the relevance of determining not only the effect of social capital on health, but also the mechanism by which this effect operates. This topic deserves more study than it has seen to date across all countries. For example two frequently mentioned mechanisms describe a positive effect of social capital on health (Folland, 2007): reduction of stress and dissemination

Table 8.2: Income per capita and health.

	High Income	Medium Income	Low Income	High/Medium Ratio	Medium/Low Ratio	High/Low Ratio
GNI per capita, PPP	32,013	9,856	1,987	3.2	5.0	16.1
All causes	10,771	19,682	34,231	0.55	0.57	0.31
Physical communicable	781	5,019	16,735	0.16	0.30	0.05
Physical non-communicable	5,953	9,006	11,371	0.66	0.80	0.53
Injuries	1,084	2,403	3,309	0.45	0.73	0.33
Neuropsychiatric (mental health)	2,952	3,254	2,870	0.91	1.13	1.03
Neuro incidence	0.28	0.19	0.10	1.50	1.85	2.78

Note: Income per capita is measured in 2004 PPP dollars. The burden of disease (by type of cause) is measured in age-standardized disability-adjusted life years (DALYs) per 100,000. Neuro incidence is the ratio of neuropsychiatric DALYs over total DALYs. Variables are averages once we segmented the 153 countries into each income group. We define as high-income countries those with GNI per capita at US$20,000 and above, as middle income countries those between US$5,000 and US$20,000, and as low-income countries those below US$5,000.
Sources: DALYs: World Health Organization (WHO), Department of Measurement and Health Information, February 2009; income per capita: World Bank.

of information. Reduction of stress indicates that a high degree of social capital decreases the perception of social isolation and may help mental health. However, it is reasonable to think that, for this mechanism to operate, the intensity of the ties may be more important than the number of social ties, and that family ties may be more effective than are ties with civic associations. The opposite may occur with the spread of information: If health information is disseminated in a social network, having a large number of weak ties may be more effective, and secondary associations' ties may be more valuable in this respect than family ties. As the number, intensity, and type of relationships evolve differently with economic development, the mechanism by which social capital affects health may also be different in developing and developed countries.

Table 8.1 shows that nuclear family ties (number and intensity) are negatively correlated with both income per capita and incidence of neuropsychiatric diseases. We also observe that the number of friends' and secondary associations' ties are positively related with both income per capita and incidence of neuropsychiatric diseases, while the intensity of friends' ties are negatively related with both. Given

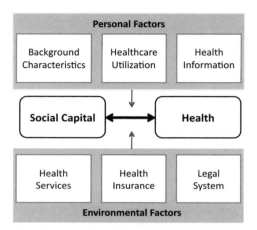

Figure 8.2: Factors that may influence social capital and health.

these observations, the main question concerns whether health effects are a direct consequence of income per capita, or are they mediated by the changes in the number, intensity, and structure of social capital. A model of the relationship between social capital, income per capita, and health is necessary to understand the causal effects between them.

There may be many pathways that link social capital and health, some of which are likely to be particularly important in low- and middle-income countries. Figure 8.2 presents a conceptual framework of personal and environmental factors that may influence the relationship between social capital and health.

Both personal factors and environmental factors are likely to influence social capital and health. Personal factors are individual characteristics, while environmental factors refer to individuals' surroundings, including the community they live in and the country's health system. Our framework highlights three personal factors that may explain the pathways in which social capital influences health: the individual's background (or demographic) characteristics, healthcare utilization, and health information.

Individual characteristics include age, gender, socio-economic status, and education, all of which are likely to be associated with individuals' levels of social capital and health. For example, Riewpaiboon *et al.* (2005) describe how social class in Thailand is linked with trust and accessibility and affordability of care, which may affect health. They find that, while inter-personal trust is important among the middle class, the Thai working class relies on impersonal trust in the hospital or health care system. Such demographic differences may mediate the relationship between social capital and health.

Health care utilization is an important pathway because social capital may affect the amount and type of care people seek, which may influence health. Trusting patients are more likely to access care at earlier phases of illness or injury, while mistrusting patients may not seek health care or may seek care only when conditions deteriorate (Goepp, 2006). In Sri Lanka, Russell (2005) finds that institutional trust, which is the basis for trust in the quality of care delivered by public providers, results in good health outcomes and that poor inter-personal relationships with public providers act as an access barrier that pushes many people to utilize the private sector. In Cambodia, Ozawa *et al.* (2011) report that trust is an important determinant of provider choice, especially for people who are seeking care from private providers. Aye *et al.* (2002) describes the critical role of social capital in the entire family's having financial access to health care services in the Ivory Coast.

Health may also affect health care utilization, which could affect social capital. The experience individuals have when seeking care may affect their trust in providers and in the health system. Health care utilization is an especially relevant link between social capital and health in low- and middle-income country contexts, where there are many barriers to accessing care and many choices between traditional (informal) and modern (formal) forms of care.

Health information could also be a vital pathway linking social capital and health. Social capital may affect the amount and types of health information to which one has access, which may affect people's care-seeking behavior and health. Individuals who are better connected in a community may have access to more sources of health information, and individuals in denser networks may be more likely to share the same health norms and health information. Edgeworth and Collins (2006) observe this mechanism in Bangladesh, where households with weaker social and human capital tended to be excluded from information on appropriate self-care treatments for diarrhea. Thiede (2005) argues that trust plays a role in the utilization of provided information, which may affect access to health care and its utilization. Since health information may be less regulated in low- and middle-income country contexts, social capital may play an important role in the health information one receives. Health can also affect the health information people receive, which could affect social capital. The health information people receive and the health care experience itself could affect their levels of trust, the information they share, and how they interact with others.

The framework also identifies three environmental factors that explain the pathway between social capital and health: health services, health insurance, and the legal system. Health services are important in explaining one of the ways in which social capital may influence health. For example, patients with more trust may be more willing than those with less trust to disclose sensitive information to physicians, allowing the physicians to provide more appropriate care and to make fewer unnecessary referrals or diagnostic tests (Thom *et al.*, 2004). Social capital may also improve the therapeutic response through better adherence to treatment, as Ware *et al.* (2009) observe in HIV/AIDS patients' adherence to anti-retroviral therapy in sub-Saharan Africa. Social capital may also improve disease surveillance through community participation, as seen in Niger (Ndiaye *et al.*, 2003).

However, it is also possible that trust in a physician leads to poorer health in some cases, as patients are less likely to seek a second opinion or to question inappropriate medical care. Benin *et al.* (2006) describe mothers who did not intend to vaccinate their children because they were unable to trust the pediatrician and who often had a trusting relationship with an influential homeopath/naturopath or other person who did not believe in vaccinating. Since health services tend to be less regulated in low- and middle-income countries, the availability and quality of treatment are likely to play a critical role in the link between social capital and health.

Health insurance could also explain the pathway that links social capital and health. Many developing countries do not have health insurance programs, and those that do exist tend to be voluntary. Individuals in communities with higher levels of social capital may have greater access to health insurance or other financial mechanisms of protection, and individuals with more social capital may be more willing to acquire health insurance, which could affect their health. Schneider (2005) finds that people in Rwanda are more likely to trust providers with good inter-personal and technical skills, and these characteristics influence individuals' enrollment decisions in micro-health insurance. Ozawa *et al.* (2011) find that, in Rwanda, people's trust in public providers and health insurers affect their decisions to enroll in a community-based health insurance programs. Zhang *et al.* (2006) find that social capital is positively associated with the probability of that farmers will be willing to join community-based health insurance programs in rural China. The importance of social capital is also described in the informal safety nets of traditional societies in Eritrea, where voluntary mutual-aid community associations and health insurance programs are built on existing social networks (Habtom and Ruys, 2007).

Social capital can affect health insurance decisions and health, and this relationship could also be reciprocal such that health affects health insurance decisions, which affect social capital. Other financing mechanisms, such as microfinance, could be pathways as well. Microcredit could affect health status by financing care and improved nutrition, providing health education, and increasing social capital through group meetings and mutual support. Schurmann *et al.* (2009) find that microcredit in Bangladesh can mitigate exclusionary processes and lead to health improvements, but it can also worsen exclusionary processes, which contribute to health disadvantage.

Finally, the legal system may also explain the pathway that links social capital and health. If the country's legal system does not protect individuals from medical errors and inappropriate care, there is a greater need for individuals to rely on social capital to make health care decisions. Riewpaiboon *et al.* (2005) report that patients in Thailand often offer a "financial incentive" to their obstetricians in hopes that they will do their best to serve the patients' best interests, although expectations were frequently not met. In Tanzania, people discussed the profit motives of private dispensaries and providers' requests for bribes as major sources of distrust (Tibandebage and Mackintosh, 2005). Khawaja *et al.* (2006) find that, while adolescents in the Palestinian refugee camp in Lebanon exhibited more social capital than those in an eastern suburb, the odds of poor health were almost four times higher for adolescents in the refugee camp. One explanation may be that the effects of legal and economic exclusion and discrimination in the refugee camp prevented Palestinian adolescents from transforming investments in social capital into individual health benefits.

In sum, there are many explanations for the relationship between social capital and health differing between developed and developing countries, including differences in the type of social capital, differences in the disease burden, and differences in the mechanisms and causal pathways that involve personal and environmental factors. The following sections shed light on these differences.

Social Capital and Health in the Developing World: Evidence in the Literature

There is widespread evidence that social capital and health are correlated in developed countries. Islam *et al.* (2006) reviews 37 studies, of which 35 were done in high-income countries and two in Russia, an upper–middle-income country.

Since the time of this review, a number of studies on the relationship between social capital and health in developing countries have been published that draw the general conclusion that there is also a strong positive association between social capital and health in these developing countries. This section of the paper reviews the evidence that supports this conclusion, considers the limitations of the evidence, and provides direction for the research needed to confirm or reject the evidence accumulated thus far.

Several studies analyze the relationship between social capital and health in developing countries, but only a few of them present causal evidence.[36] D'Hombres et al. (2010) and Ronconi et al. (2012) use instrumental variables to address the problems of endogeneity and reverse causation. D'Hombres et al. (2010) find that higher degrees of trust and lower degrees of social isolation positively affect health in eight transition countries that were part of the former Soviet Union. Ronconi et al. (2012) show that interactions with family and friends in Argentina have a positive effect on health. To date, there is no causal evidence that suggests that secondary associations affect health positively in developing countries.

A much larger set of studies shows the relationship between social capital and health rather than causation, and some of which analyze dimensions of the correlation between social capital and health. Using a rich dataset of Russians, Rose (2000) shows that some measures of social capital (i.e., trust and the presence of someone to rely on when one is ill) are positively associated with better physical and emotional health, but those who rely on friends for information have worse physical and emotional health. Some of these rich datasets could be used to infer the size and mechanisms of the effects. Social capital (friends) may act positively on health through providing support when one is ill but not through information diffusion. The strongest association is between the perception of having control over one's life and health, but it is not clear whether the variable (having control over one's life) is a good measure of social capital.

Poortinga (2006) uses individual data for 22 high- and middle-income European countries to find a strong association between individual measures of trust and civic participation and self-rated health, while equivalent aggregate variables are

---

[36]Other analyses of the relationship between social capital and health in developing countries includes that of De Silva et al. (2007), Mansyur et al. (2008), Hurtado et al. (2011), Harpham et al. (2004), Surkan et al. (2009), Bakeera (2010), and Elgar et al. (2011).

generally not associated with individual health. However, Poortinga suggests a difference between societies with high social capital and those with low social capital: Individuals with high social capital in countries characterized by high social capital have better health than those who have low social capital, but the same cannot be said for countries with low social capital. This finding suggests that, for example, trusting is beneficial for the health of a person if a majority of the society in which he lives is also trusting, while it may not be so if the majority of the group is distrustful. This suggestion points to a positive externality of social capital and to a coordination problem in its provision.

Baron-Epel *et al.* (2008) obtain a similar result in a study of the relationship between social capital and health in Israel, separating Jews from Arabs. The authors find a positive association between most measures of social capital (including trust and social support) and self-rated health for Jews, who show high aggregate levels of social capital, but the association is inexistent or weak for Arabs, who show low aggregate levels of social capital.

Ferlander *et al.* (2009) obtain weaker results in a study of Moscovites, showing that the association between self-related health and social capital, measured by frequency of visits to relatives and friends and by participation in civic associations, is significant for men but not for women. Rojas and Carlson (2006) use a survey of individuals in Taganrog, Russia to find that being a member of an organization (which they separate into trade unions or political organizations and "any other organization") is positively related to self-reported health. When they interact these variables with the level of education, a subtler picture appears: Participating in trade unions or political organizations is beneficial for less educated individuals, while participating in other types of organizations is beneficial for highly educated individuals.

Wang *et al.* (2009) examine self-reported health and social capital as measured by inter-personal trust and mistrust in rural China, observing that only when personal trust levels reach a certain point does social capital begin to be associated with health. Mistrust effects are generally more pronounced at the individual level, while trust effects are more pronounced at the village level. One of the results is an unexpected protective health effect of mistrust in certain villages.

All in all, there is strong evidence of a positive association between some forms of social capital and some measures of health in developing countries and some preliminary evidence of a causal link between some forms of social capital and some measures of health. Moreover, there is evidence that individual social capital is more strongly associated with health than is community-level social capital. Still, aggregate social capital seems to play a role in determining the strength of the association between individual social capital and health.

Two issues should be analyzed more in depth in future research. First, the mechanisms by which certain forms of social capital affect health should be analyzed more thoroughly and explicitly explained. A good example of research that is well analyzed and explained is Yamamura's (2011) study of the relationship between social capital and health in Japan. The study discriminated between workers and non-workers based on the hypothesis that non-workers should present a stronger relationship between neighborhood associations and health because the opportunity cost of investing in that type of social capital is lower for them than for workers. The study then provides evidence supporting the hypothesis by showing the association between the variables and giving some evidence of causality with suitable instrumental variables.

Second, too little attention has been given to Durlauf's (2002) critiques and suggestions: Durlauf suggests that, "in using observational studies, it seems clear that researchers need to provide explicit models of the co-determination of individual outcomes and social capital." However, none of the studies reviewed on the relationship between social capital and health in developing countries presents such a model. Durlauf also encourages the use of economic experiments of the type conducted by social psychologists: "The design of the experiment renders inoperative worries about omitted control variables, differences between groups, etc.," but we find no such experiment to address the question of the relationship between social capital and health in developing countries.

Further Evidence

Beyond these concerns, because of differences in data, measurement, and methodology, available evidence does not allow the size of the effects of social capital on health to be compared across countries. This is a major limitation when analyzing the three-way relationship among social capital, health, and development, as it does not permit testing for whether the effects of social capital on health are larger or smaller in developing compared to developed countries, or the analysis of whether different types of social capital have different effects on health depending on the level of economic development.

In this section we compute and compare country estimates using a homogenous database of 34 countries (included in ISSP, 2007). The survey is particularly useful for our purposes because it includes three alternative measures of social capital (i.e., informal social interactions, participation in organizations, and trust), and it was conducted in countries with different levels of economic development, including 24 high-income countries, nine upper–middle-income countries, and one lower–middle-income country (the Philippines). No low-income country is represented in the dataset.[37] We also explore variations in the relationship between social capital and health across regions in Argentina, an upper–middle-income country with large disparities in the level of development across provinces.

Comparison across countries

The ISSP dataset shows that trust and participation in organizations are higher in developed countries and that countries with higher income have lower levels of social interactions with friends and family (see Figures 8.3 to 8.5). Similar results are reported by Anchorena and Anjos (2008).

To determine whether the social capital effects on health differ by level of economic development, we first compute estimates by region and country and then compare them across countries with similar cultural or institutional characteristics. The statistical model is:

$$Health_{ij} = \beta_1 InformalSK_{ij} + \beta_2 ParticipationSK_{ij} + \beta_3 Trust_{ij} + \delta X_{ij} + \varepsilon_{ij}$$

$$(8.1)$$

where $Health_{ij}$ is a self-assessed categorical variable that takes values from 1 to 5 (1 = excellent, 5 = poor) for individual i in country j; and X includes sex, age, education, family size, and family income. We treat self-rated health as a continuous variable and estimate Eq. (8.1) using OLS.[38]

---

[37]The countries in the ISSP 2007 are Argentina, Australia, Austria, Belgium, Bulgaria, Chile, Croatia, Cyprus, the Czech Republic, the Dominican Republic, Finland, France, Germany, Great Britain, Hungary, Ireland, Israel, Japan, Latvia, Mexico, New Zealand, Norway, the Philippines, Poland, Russia, Slovakia, Slovenia, South Africa, South Korea, Sweden, Switzerland, Taiwan, the United States, and Uruguay.

[38]The model we estimate suffers from some of the identification problems described in the previous section, so the estimates we compute are likely to be biased. However, there is no reason to think *a priori* that those biases differ across countries.

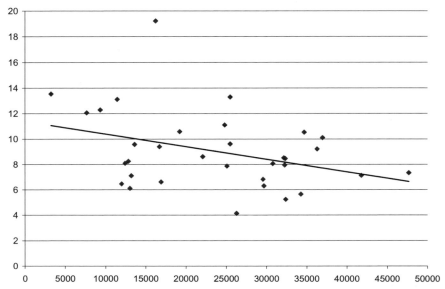

Figure 8.3: Informal social interactions (frequency of meeting with friends per month) and GDP per capita across countries in 2007.

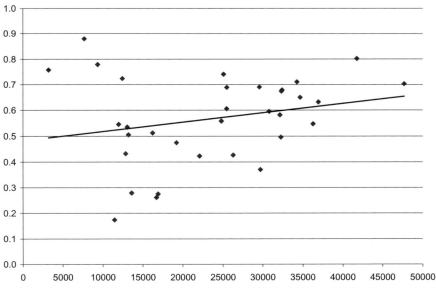

Figure 8.4: Participation in organizations (share of the population that participates) and GDP per capita across countries in 2007.

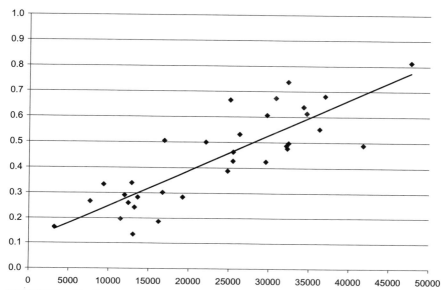

Figure 8.5: Trust (share of the population that trusts other people) and GDP per capita across countries in 2007.

We first divide the sample into five groups (developed countries, Latin America, Eastern Europe, South Africa, and the Philippines) and compute estimates for each group using Eq. (8.1), including country fixed-effects except when the sample is restricted to single countries, such as is the case with South Africa and the Philippines (Table 8.3). We find that both participation in organizations and trust are negatively correlated with health problems in all regions, but the variable of informal interactions affects health only in Latin America. With the exception of the coefficient for trust, which appears to have a larger impact in more developed regions, there is no evidence that the magnitude of the coefficients is correlated with the level of development.

The estimates in Table 8.3 could be capturing some common cultural or institutional factors within the region, so we estimate country coefficients and compare them across countries within the same region (Table 8.4). Because Eastern Europe contains countries that differ significantly in their levels of development, this is an interesting region to explore. We find that informal social capital is not significantly correlated with health in any country except the Slovak Republic, where it has the opposite effect. On the other hand, trust is negatively correlated with health problems, as expected, in every country, and participation in organizations

Table 8.3: Estimates of the effect of social capital on health by region.

Region	GDP pc	Informal SC	Participation SC	Trust
Developed	32,541	−0.02	−0.14***	−0.20***
Eastern Europe	17,119	0.01	−0.12***	−0.15***
Latin America	11,665	−0.05***	−0.05*	−0.12***
South Africa	9,333	−0.01	−0.15**	−0.06***
Philippines	3,216	0.05	−0.19**	−0.11**

Note: The dependent variable is self-assessed health problems. "GDPpc" stands for per capita gross domestic product and "SC" for social capital. Column (1) presents the average GDP per capita in 2009 in the region (PPP constant 2005 international US dollars). Columns (2), (3), and (4) present the coefficients for informal social interactions, participation in organizations, and trust, respectively. Each row is a different regression. Estimates are computed including country dummies and clustering the standard errors (omitted) by country. *Significant at the $p = 0.1$, **0.05, and ***0.01 levels.

Table 8.4: Country estimates of the effect of social capital on health in Eastern Europe.

Country	GDP pc	Informal SC	Participation SC	Trust
Slovenia	24,807	0.08	−0.07	−0.22***
Czech Republic	22,098	0.04	−0.14**	−0.15***
Slovak Republic	19,202	0.08**	−0.07	−0.20***
Poland	16,705	−0.04	0.03	−0.14***
Croatia	16,225	0.05	0.02	−0.17***
Russia	13,611	0.02	−0.13***	−0.11***
Latvia	12,849	−0.03	−0.17***	−0.20***
Bulgaria	11,458	0.03	−0.11	−0.13***

Note: The dependent variable is self-assessed health problems. Column (1) presents GDP per capita. Columns (2), (3), and (4) present the coefficients for informal social interactions, participation in organizations, and trust, respectively. Each row is a different regression. Robust standard errors (omitted). *Significant at the $p = 0.1$, **0.05, and ***0.01 levels.

is negatively correlated with health in most countries. We observe no evidence suggesting that the magnitude of the coefficients depends on the level of economic development. For example, trust has a large effect on health in Slovenia, a high-income country in the OECD, as well as in Latvia, an upper–middle-income country.

In the sample of Latin American countries included in the ISSP survey, there is also some variation in levels of economic development (Table 8.5). We find that

Table 8.5: Country estimates of the effect of social capital on health in Latin America.

Country	GDP pc	Informal SC	Participation SC	Trust
Argentina	13,202	−0.06***	−0.01	−0.12***
Chile	13,057	−0.03	−0.10	−0.16***
Mexico	12,429	−0.03	−0.16**	−0.18***
Uruguay	11,977	−0.02	−0.14***	−0.05
Dominican Rep.	7,658	−0.06**	0.10	−0.11***

Note: The dependent variable is self-assessed health problems. Column (1) presents GDP per capita. Columns (2), (3), and (4) present the coefficients for informal social interactions, participation in organizations, and trust, respectively. Each row is a different regression. Robust standard errors (omitted). *Significant at the $p = 0.1$, **0.05, and ***0.01 levels.

informal social capital, participation in organizations, and trust are, as expected, negatively and significantly correlated with health problems but no evidence that the level of development is correlated with the size of the coefficients.

Table 8.6 presents estimates for the remaining countries in the survey, which are all relatively rich. Informal social capital is not significantly correlated with health in any of the countries with the exception of Cyprus and Ireland (with the expected sign) and Germany and Israel (with the contrary sign). On the other hand, participation in organizations and trust are significantly correlated with health in most of the countries.

Finally, Figure 8.6 plots the estimated country coefficients and GDP per capita.[39] There is a statistically significant association between GDP per capita and the effect of trust on health; that is, in richer countries an increase in trust has a larger protective effect on health. There is no clear relationship between the size of estimated coefficients for the other two measures of social capital (informal interactions and participation in organizations) and GDP per capita.

In sum, the cross-country comparison suggests that people in more developed countries have higher levels of trust, higher levels of participation in organizations, and fewer interactions with friends and family. In addition, the country estimates indicate that individuals who have more trust and higher levels of participation in organizations tend to have better health, a result observed in the majority of

---

[39]We assume a coefficient of zero for the two countries (Austria and Uruguay) where trust has no statistically significant effect on health.

Table 8.6: Country estimates of the effect of social capital on health, developed countries.

Country	GDP pc	Informal SC	Participation SC	Trust
Norway	47,676	0.05	−0.28***	−0.13***
United States	41,761	0.01	−0.16**	−0.27***
Switzerland	36,954	−0.01	−0.16**	−0.17***
Ireland	36,278	−0.07*	−0.07	−0.23***
Austria	34,673	0.07	−0.13*	−0.05
Australia	34,259	0.01	−0.04	−0.20***
Belgium	32,395	−0.05	−0.18**	−0.14***
Sweden	32,314	0.04	−0.06	−0.17***
Germany	32,255	0.06*	−0.08	−0.16***
Great Britain	32,147	0.03	−0.18**	−0.17***
Finland	30,784	0.05	−0.14**	−0.17***
Japan	29,692	0.01	−0.14**	−0.30***
France	29,578	0.01	0.04	−0.21***
Cyprus	26,373	−0.05***	−0.11**	−0.15***
South Korea	25,493	−0.01	−0.09	−0.13***
Israel	25,474	0.09***	−0.18***	−0.16***
New Zealand	25,088	0.04	−0.07	−0.21***

Note: The dependent variable is self-assessed health problems. Column (1) presents GDP per capita. Columns (2), (3), and (4) present the coefficients for informal social interactions, participation in organizations, and trust, respectively. Each row is a different regression. Robust standard errors (omitted). *Significant at the $p = 0.1$, **0.05 and ***0.01 levels.

countries. There is some evidence that people who interact more frequently with friends have better health, but this result is observed primarily in Latin America. Finally, the size of trust's effect on health is larger in more developed countries than in less developed ones. Combining all of these results, we conclude that the better health outcomes observed in more developed countries occur in part because their populations have more trust and participation in organizations and because of a larger effect of trust on health.

Why does trust have a larger "return" in richer countries? We speculate that one explanation is the positive relationship between economic development and the incidence of mental health relative to physical health problems. If trust reduces stress and, as a result, mental health problems, then it should have a larger effect on health in those countries where mental illness is more prevalent than in those where it is less prevalent.

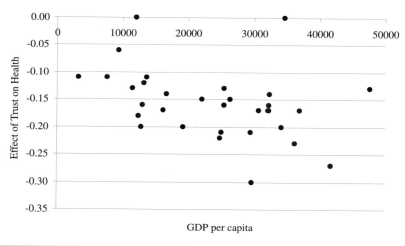

Figure 8.6: The effects of trust on health across levels of development.

Comparison across regions within a country

In this section we study the case of Argentina, a country with large disparities in economic development across regions. We categorize provinces according to the level of economic development in three groups: the relatively rich, which includes those jurisdictions with income per capita above US$6,000 per year in 1997 (i.e., City of Buenos Aires, Chubut, Santa Cruz and Tierra del Fuego); the relatively poor, which includes those with income per capita below US$3,000 per year (i.e., Corrientes, Formosa, Jujuy, Salta and Santiago del Estero), and those in between.

We use a household survey, the Social Development Survey, which provides measures of interactions with friends and family, participation in organizations, and health, although the survey does not include a measure of trust. We use the same data and variable definitions as Ronconi *et al.* (2012) use and compute estimates for each region using the following statistical model:

$$Health\ Problem_i = \mu_1 InformalSK_i + \mu_2 ParticipationSK_i + \theta X_i + \varepsilon_i \quad (8.2)$$

where the dependent variable is a self-assessed binary variable ($1=$ individual i reports health problems, $0 =$ no health problems); X includes sex, age, education, family size, and income. We estimate Eq. (8.2) using a probit model.

Table 8.7: *Estimates of the effect of social capital on health across regions in Argentina.*

Region	Informal SC	Participation SC
Richest provinces	−0.09***	0.05
Middle income provinces	−0.08***	−0.01
Poorest provinces	−0.11***	−0.03**

Note: The dependent variable is a self-assessed binary variable that indicates health problems. Column (1) presents the coefficients for informal social interactions and column (2) presents those for participation in organizations. Each row is a different regression. Robust standard errors (omitted). *Significant at the $p = 0.1$, **0.05, and ***0.01 levels.

We find that, in all regions of Argentina, people with more interactions with friends and family are less likely to report health problems and that the estimates are of similar magnitude across regions with different levels of economic development. On the other hand, we find evidence of a negative correlation between participation in organizations and health problems in the less developed provinces (Table 8.7). These results are consistent with those obtained using the ISSP dataset. Lack of information on trust precludes testing whether the relationship between the size of the estimated effects of trust and GDP per capita observed across countries also occurs across regions within Argentina.

Summary and Concluding Remarks

This chapter posits a series of questions related to the trio of social capital, health, and economic development; reviews the empirical literature of social capital and health in developing countries; and uses a homogenous international dataset, the International Social Survey Programme (ISSP), to computes new estimates that exploit variations across countries and variation within regions in Argentina. The main conclusion drawn in the chapter is that social capital is positively correlated with better health outcomes in the developing world, and that some studies show that there is also a causal relationship. More tentatively, we conclude that — with the exception of trust, which has a larger return on in more developed countries — the magnitude of the effects does not vary with the level of economic development.

The study leads to several directions for further research. First, future research should distinguish between different forms of social capital and kinds of health problems. These distinctions are particularly important, given that countries with higher levels of economic development tend to have more trust, more participation in organizations, and fewer family ties but also a lower incidence of physical health problems, with the exception of mental health. We lack information about the dynamic relationships among these factors.

Second, the large majority of applied research has focused on computing correlations between social capital and health, a useful first step. However, theory suggests that not only does social capital affect health but health affects social capital. Further analysis based on experimental evidence would be particularly valuable.

Finally, the mechanisms by which specific forms of social capital affect different types of health problems and how these mechanisms depend on institutional factors deserve more attention.

References

Anchorena, J. and Anjos, F. 2008. Social ties and economic development. Ph.D thesis, Carnegie Mellon University.

Arrow, K. 2000. Observations on social capital. In *Social Capital: A Multifaceted Perspective*, eds. Dasgupta, P. and Serageldin, I, pp. 3–5. The World Bank, Washington DC.

Aye, M., Champagne, F. and Contandriopoulos. A. 2002. Economic role of solidarity and social capital in accessing modern health care services in the Ivory Coast. *Social Science and Medicine*, 55: 1929–1946.

Bakeera, S. K., Petzold, M., Pariyo, G. W., Galea, S., Tomson, G. and Wamala, S. 2010. Community social capital and the use of health care services in Uganda. *Journal of Public Health and Epidemiology*, 2(8): 189–198.

Baron-Epel, O., Garty-Sandalon, N., Green, M. S., Haviv-Mesika, A. and Weinstein, R. 2008. Individual-level analysis of social capital and health: A comparison of Arab and Jewish Israelis. *Social Science and Medicine*, 66(4): 900–910.

Benin, A. L., Wisler-Scher, D. J., Colson, E., Shapiro, E. D. and Holmboe, E. S. 2006. Qualitative analysis of mothers' decision-making about vaccines for infants: The importance of trust. *Pediatrics*, 117(5): 1532–1541.

Carlson, P. and Rojas, Y. 2006. The stratification of social capital and its consequences for self-rated health in Taganrog, Russia. *Social Science and Medicine*, 62(11): 2732–2741.

Coleman, J. S. 1988. Social capital in the creation of human capital. *The American Journal of Sociology*, 94: 95–120.

De Silva, M., Huttly, S., Harpham, T. and Kenward, M. 2007. Social capital and mental health: A comparative analysis of four low income countries. *Social Science and Medicine*, 64(1): 5–20.

d'Hombres, B., Rocco, L., Suhrcke, M. and McKee, M. 2010. Does social capital determine health? Evidence from eight transition countries. *Health Economics*, 19(1): 56–74.

Durlauf, S. N. 2002. On the empirics of social capital. *The Economic Journal*, 112(483): F459–F479.

Edgeworth, R. and Collins, A. 2006. Self-care as a response to diarrhoea in rural Bangladesh: Empowered choice or enforced adoption? *Social Science and Medicine*, 63: 2686–2897.

Elgar, F. J. and Aitken, N. 2010. Income inequality, trust and homicide in 33 countries. *European Journal of Public Health*, 21(2): 241–246.

Ferlander, S. and Mäkinen, I. H. 2009. Social capital, gender and self-rated health. Evidence from the Moscow Health Survey 2004. *Social Science and Medicine*, 69(9): 1323–1332.

Folland, S. 2007. Does "community social capital" contribute to population health? *Social Science and Medicine*, 64(11): 2342–2354.

Goepp, J. G. 2006. Reflections on trust and health services utilization. *Preventive Medicine*, 42: 81–82.

Guiso, L., Sapienza, P. and Zingales, L. 2004. The role of social capital in financial development. *American Economic Review*, 94: 526–556.

Habtom, G. K. and Ruys, P. 2007. Traditional risk-sharing arrangements and informal social insurance in Eritrea. *Health Policy*, 80(1): 218–235.

Harpham, T., Grant, E. and Rodriguez, C. 2004. Mental health and social capital in Cali, Colombia. *Social Science and Medicine*, 58(11): 2267–2277.

Hurtado, D., Kawachi, I. and Sudarsky, J. 2011. Social capital and self-rated health in Colombia: The good, the bad and the ugly. *Social Science and Medicine*, 72(4): 584–590.

Islam M. K., Merlo, J., Kawachi, I., Lindström, M. and Gerdtham, G. 2007. Social capital and health: Does egalitarianism matter? A literature review. *International Journal for Equity in Health*, 5: 3.

Khawaja, M., Abdulrahim, S., Soweid, R. A. and Karam, D. 2006. Distrust, social fragmentation and adolescents' health in the outer city: Beirut and beyond. *Social Science and Medicine*, 63: 1304–1315.

Mansyur, C., Amick, B. C., Harrist, R. B. and Franzini, L. 2007. Social capital, income inequality, and self-rated health in 45 countries. *Social Science and Medicine*, 66(1): 43–56.

Ndiaye, S., Quick, L., Sanda, O. and Niandou, S. 2003. The value of community participation in disease surveillance: A case study from Niger. *Health Promotion International*, 18(2): 89–98.

Ozawa, S. and Walker, D. 2011. Comparison of trust in public vs private health care providers in rural Cambodia. *Health Policy and Planning*, 26: i20–i29.

Poortinga, W. 2006. Social relations or social capital? Individual and community health effects of bonding social capital. *Social Science and Medicine*, 66(1): 43–56.

Riewpaiboon, W., Chuengsatiansup, K., Gilson, L. and Tangcharoensathien, V. 2005. Private obstetric practice in public hospital: Mythical trust in obstetric care. *Social Science and Medicine*, 61: 1408–1417.

Rojas, Y. and Carlson, P. 2006. The stratification of social capital and its consequences for self-rated health in Taganrog, Russia. *Social Science and Medicine*, 62(1): 2732–2741.

Ronconi, L., Brown, T. and Sheffler, R. 2012. Social capital and self-rated health in Argentina. *Health Economics*, 21(2): 201–208.

Rose, R. 2000. How much does social capital add to individual health? A survey study of Russians. *Social Science and Medicine*, 51(9): 1421–1435.

Russell, S. 2005. Treatment-seeking behavior in urban Sri Lanka: Trusting the state, trusting private providers. *Social Science and Medicine*, 61: 1396–1407.

Schneider, P. 2005. Trust in micro-health insurance: An exploratory study in Rwanda. *Social Science and Medicine*, 61(7): 1430–1438.

Schurmann, A., and Johnston, H. 2009. The group-lending model and social closure: Microcredit, exclusion, and health in Bangladesh. *Journal of Health Population and Nutrition*, 27(4): 518–527.

Solow, R. 2000. Notes on social capital and economic performance. In *Social Capital: A Multifaceted Perspective*, eds., Dasgupta, P. and Serageldin, I., pp. 6–10. The World Bank, Washington DC.

Surkan, P. J., O'Donnell, E., Berkman, L. and Peterson, K. E. 2010. Social ties in relation to health status of low-income Brazilian women. *Journal of Women's Health*, 18(12): 2049–2056.

Thiede, M. 2005. Information and access to health care: Is there a role for trust? *Social Science and Medicine*, 61: 1452–1462.

Thom, D. H., Hall, M. A. and Pawlson, L. G. 2004. Measuring patients' trust in physicians when assessing quality of care. *Health Affairs*, 23(4): 124–132.

Tibandebage, P. and Mackintosh, M. 2005. The market shaping of charges, trust and abuse: Health care transactions in Tanzania. *Social Science and Medicine*, 61(7): 1385–1395.

Yamamura, E. 2011. Differences in the effect of social capital on health status between workers and non-workers. *International Review of Economics*, 58(4): 385–400.

Wang, Hongmei, Schlesinger, M., Wang, H. and Hsiao, W. 2009. The flip-side of social capital: The distinctive influences of trust and mistrust on health in rural China. *Social Science and Medicine*, 68: 133–142.

Ware, N., Idoko, J., Kaaya, S., Biraro, I., Wyatt, M., Agbaji, O., Chalamilla, G. and Bangsberg, D. 2009. Explaining adherence success in sub-Saharan Africa: An ethnographic study. *PLoS Medicine*, 6(1): e1000011.

Zhang, L., Wang, H., Wang, L. and Hsiao, W. 2006. Social capital and farmer's willingness-to-join a newly established community-based health insurance in rural China. *Health Policy*, 76(2): 233–242.

Chapter 9

Social Capital and Smoking

Lorenzo Rocco and Beatrice d'Hombres

Introduction

The analysis of the relationship between social capital and smoking, and more generally between social capital and health-related behaviors, has been the only attempt to study a specific pathway through which social capital influences individual health. Health-related behaviors, critical inputs for individual health, may convey a substantial part of the overall beneficial influence of social capital on health. However, although the literature generally suggests that higher levels of social capital lead to more responsible health-related behaviors (Lindström, 2003; Lundborg, 2005), the mechanisms at work behind this relationship — *why* social capital leads to more responsible behaviors — remain unclear. Only reduced-form models have been estimated in the empirical literature, with the majority of studies being devoted to the relationship between social capital and smoking or social capital and alcohol and/or cannabis use.

This chapter goes beyond reduced forms to explore one mechanism that may underlie the negative relationship between social capital and smoking behavior. Specifically, we want to test whether social capital does strengthen the compliance to anti-smoking regulations. The purpose of government-imposed smoking bans is to reduce the negative externalities associated with smoking by protecting the public from environmental tobacco smoke ("second-hand smoke"). Since smokers who have high levels of social capital are more likely to internalize the private and social costs of their behaviors, they should comply more strictly with the smoking ban regulation than would those with less social capital.

To determine whether these bans' impact on smoking prevalence and intensity is larger among individuals with high levels of social capital, we use data collected immediately before and immediately after the implementation of smoking bans in public places in Germany between 2007 and 2008.

Germany, like many other European countries, recently introduced the prohibition of smoking in government buildings, bars, restaurants, and dance clubs. Although smoking in public places is now prohibited nationwide, the date on which the ban was introduced was left partly to the discretion of each state, so it took effect at various times between October 2007 and July 2008.

We use the German Socio-Economic Panel (SOEP) for the empirical analysis. This representative household panel survey is particularly suitable in our context, as it includes information on both smoking behaviors and social capital. In order to identify the effect of the smoking ban we exploit a peculiar feature of the SOEP, namely the fact that respondents are contacted and interviewed continuously between February and October. Therefore, in the German states that enacted their bans between February and October of 2008, we observe a sample of individuals interviewed just before the introduction of the ban and other respondents interviewed just after. Since the date of the interview depends essentially on organizational reasons and is likely to be orthogonal to individual characteristics like smoking and individual social capital, we have a quasi-experimental framework that involves a random assignment to treatment and control groups, with the treatment group being those people who were interviewed after the introduction of the smoking ban, and the control group being those interviewed before. Therefore, a simple-difference model that compares smoking prevalence and intensity between the treatment group and the control group, conditioning on state fixed-effects, can be used to evaluate the impact of smoking bans. Moreover, since German states introduced the ban at various times, we can account for the seasonal effects that might influence smoking behavior.

Within this framework, the investigation of whether impacts of the smoking ban differ based on the level of individual social capital is relatively straightforward. First, we show that interacting the treatment indicator with one social capital indicator will provide unbiased estimates of the differential effect that is due to social capital, even if the latter is endogenous. Next, we select three complementary measures of social capital — two related to individual trust and one related to participation in volunteer activities — to investigate the interaction between smoking bans and social capital.

We find that the German smoking bans reduced both smoking prevalence and intensity, at least among men, and that individual social capital strengthens personal compliance with smoking bans. The probability that men who report a higher level of trust would smoke fell by about 6 percent after the introduction of the smoking ban, while we saw no effect for their less trusting counterparts. Among the male smokers, the number of cigarettes smoked per day decreased by about five units among the more trusting men, while there was no reduction among the less trusting men. We find less precise estimates, although they point in the same direction, when we use participation in volunteer activities as a measure of social capital.

The rest of the analysis is organized as follows: We first discuss the literature most related to this study. We then describe the process of introducing smoking bans in Germany, followed by the data and definitions of our social capital measures. The next section explains in detail our identification strategy and the specification of the empirical model. Results are discussed and we conclude the chapter with some remarks.

Literature Review

Several mechanisms have been proposed to rationalize the negative effect of social capital on smoking prevalence and intensity (Lindström, 2008; Lundborg, 2005; Lindström, 2003). One of the proposed mechanisms is that, by favoring more intense and frequent social interactions, social capital supports the creation of information channels and helps to spread public health campaign messages, strategies for smoking cessation, and information about the dangers of tobacco. Another is that social capital can enhance trust in the public and governmental institutions that are usually in charge of delivering anti-smoking campaigns. Along these lines, Lindström (2003) suggests that people with a low level of trust are less likely to respond to doctors' advice and recommendations or to be influenced by anti-smoking public health campaigns. Yet another proposed mechanism is that communities rich in social capital may be keener than other communities to impose and enforce norms and sanctions against smoking in order to reduce the negative externalities that result from smoking. If we extend social capital to civic capital (Guiso *et al.*, 2010), then people who are more civic-minded tend to obey regulations because they understand and value the socially positive effect of doing so. It is this last mechanism that we scrutinize in this work.

Rather than providing a comprehensive review of the literature on the relationship between social capital and health-related behaviors — we refer the reader to Lindström (2008) for a complete and accurate review — we focus on a limited number of innovative studies for their underlying economic model and/or empirical strategy.

Since smoking negatively affects individual probability of survival, Folland *et al.* (2011) note that the utility loss that is due to smoking increases as the expected utility that can be enjoyed in the future increases. As investments in social capital increase future utility, especially when exogenously given social conditions enable high returns on these investments, there would be a negative relationship between individual social capital and smoking. Folland and colleagues confirm this theoretical prediction using Norwegian data and instrumenting social capital with its lagged value.

Brown *et al.* (2011) assume that social capital increases the individual perception of the harmful effect of smoking, thereby altering the opportunity costs of smoking. Brown and colleagues adapted their model from Folland (2006) and tested it using data from California. The authors instrument community social capital, measured by the Petris Index, with weather characteristics and ethnic heterogeneity at the county level in California and find that social capital significantly reduces smoking.

Several studies report negative associations between social capital and smoking in various countries and settings. Tampubolon *et al.* (2011) use a path multi-level analysis to conclude that community (structural) social capital is negatively associated with smoking in Wales. Li and Delva (2011, 2012) find that individual measures of cognitive social capital are associated with less smoking among Asian Americans and that measures of structural social capital have no association with smoking. Similarly, Takakura (2011) finds that measures of individual cognitive social capital (trust and reciprocity) are negatively associated with smoking among Japanese students between the ages of 15 and 18. Lindström (2009) reports that, in southern Sweden, people with low levels of political trust and low levels generalized trust in other people are more likely to be daily smokers than are those who have high levels of such trust.[40]

---

[40]The seminal early studies on this topic are Lundborg (2005), which finds a negative correlation between individual social capital (trust and social participation) and drinking

Several papers have questioned the effect of smoking bans in Europe. Origo and Lucifora (2010) conduct a cross-country analysis to study the impact of the introduction of smoking bans on workers' perceptions of their health and the presence of respiratory problems in the workplace. They use the variation in the timing of the introduction of smoking bans in European countries to identify the effect by means of a difference-in-differences strategy. Jones *et al.* (2011) evaluate the impact of a smoking ban introduction on smoking propensity and intensity in the UK, where the timing of introduction was not uniform between England and Scotland, allowing for difference-in-differences and change-in-changes identification strategies. They find that the introduction of the smoking ban in the UK had no impact on overall smoking prevalence but that it led to a reduction in the daily consumption of cigarettes, especially among male heavy smokers, female moderate and heavy smokers, and young people.

Anger *et al.* (2011) follow an analogous strategy, using the variation in the timing of ban introduction among German states between 2007 and 2008, to conclude, similar to Jones *et al.* (2011), that the introduction of smoke-free legislation in Germany did not change average smoking behavior. However they find that individuals who often go out to bars and restaurants smoke less after the ban than they did before it. In this chapter we use the same data set used by Anger *et al.* (2011), but our empirical identification strategy differs from theirs. In addition, unlike Anger *et al.* (2011), we specifically test to determine whether social capital affects the impact of smoke-free-air legislation on smoking behaviors. Using Italian data, Buonanno and Ranzani (2012) independently adopt an approach similar to ours and find that the smoking regulation introduced in Italy in 2005 led to a decline in smoking prevalence and intensity in both men and women.

Smoking Regulation in Germany

Several complementary tobacco control measures have been adopted in Germany in recent years. While the cost of cigarettes remained stable in the 1970s, 1980s,

---

and smoking among Swedish adolescents aged 12–18, and Lindström (2003), which shows that daily smoking in Sweden is negatively associated with both social participation and trust, while intermittent smoking is positively associated with social participation and negatively associated with trust.

and 1990s, the years since 1999 have seen several excise increases, with significant effects on the real price of cigarettes (Göhlmann and Schmidt, 2008). Since 2007, considerable emphasis has been placed on curtailing youth smoking and exposure to second-hand smoke. Since January 2007 vending machines have had to be equipped with devices for electronic age verification, and in September 2007 the federal legal minimum smoking age increased from 16 to 18 for vending machines the new legal age has been enforced only since January 2009 — and smoking bans in federal buildings, train stations, and public transport were introduced. Finally, between August 2007 and July 2008 smoking bans in public places were enacted in all German states (Kvasnicka, 2010).

This chapter focuses on the last regulatory intervention because smoking bans, much more than taxation or sales restrictions, have a role in countering second-hand smoke, the negative externality associated with individual smoking, where social capital might play a role. We also choose this regulation because smoking bans at the state level were introduced at various times, allowing for a clearer identification of their effects.

The decision to ban smoking in public places was made in early 2007 at a conference of all state health ministers, but it was left to the states to devise and enact the bans. Baden–Wurttemberg and Lower Saxony were the first (both in August 2007) to impose smoking bans in public places, and North-Rhine Westphalia and Thuringia were the last (in July 2008). As Table 9.1 shows, the date of introduction sometimes differed from the date on which violations were first fined, so in the empirical analysis, we consider the latter as the relevant date of introduction of the smoking ban. With the exception of Bavaria, all states allowed pubs and restaurants to operate separating smoking rooms, and the majority of the states also allowed dance clubs to have smoking rooms. Since small single-room establishments could not, by definition, have a separate smoking room, this rule was considered unfair to small establishments and the Federal Constitutional Court ruled in July 2008 that smoking in single-room establishments was to be allowed until the end of 2009, and that bars smaller than 75 square meters were allowed to declare themselves "smoking pubs" only if people under the age of 19 were denied entry and food was not served. The majority of states followed the Constitutional Court's ruling by adding this exemption clause to their state smoking ban legislation (Anger *et al.*, 2011).

Table 9.1: State smoking bans: introduction, fining of violations, and exemptions.

Federal States	State Smoking Bans		Smoking Rooms Permissible in:	
	Introduction	Fining of Violations	Bars/ Restaurants	Clubs
Baden–Wurttemberg	2007/08/01	at once	yes	yes
Bavaria	2008/01/01	at once	no	no
Berlin	2008/01/01	2008/07/01	yes	yes
Brandenburg	2008/01/01	2008/07/01	yes	no
Bremen	2008/01/01	2008/07/01	yes	yes
Hamburg	2008/01/01	at once	yes	yes
Hesse	2007/10/01	at once	yes	yes
Lower Saxony	2007/08/01	2007/11/01	yes	no
Mecklenburg West-Pomerania	2008/01/01	2008/08/01	yes	no
North Rhine-Westphalia	2008/07/01	at once	yes	yes
Rhineland-Palatinate	2008/02/15	at once	yes	yes
Saarland	2008/02/15	2008/06/01	yes	yes
Saxony	2008/02/01	at once	yes	no
Saxony-Anhalt	2008/01/01	2008/07/01	yes	no
Schleswig-Holstein	2008/01/01	at once	yes	yes
Thuringia	2008/07/01	at once	yes	yes

Source: Michael Kvasnicka (2010) based on information collected from original law texts and from a survey of state-level smoking ban legislation by the German Hotels and Restaurants Federation (DEHOGA, 2008).

Data

Our empirical analysis is based on the German Socio-Economic Panel (SOEP),[41] a representative household survey collected by the German Institute for Economic Research (DIW). Since 1984, around 20,000 individuals have been interviewed every year on a wide range of issues related to their socio-economic conditions. In particular, the SOEP collects information on educational, working, and income conditions and health status, including smoking behavior. In some waves, such as in 2008, questions related to social capital are also asked.

---

[41] See Wagner *et al.* (2007) for additional information about the SOEP.

In this chapter we use data from the 2006 and 2008 waves. (The 2007 wave does not report data on smoking.) An important feature of the SOEP data collection process is that it takes place from February to October, and the precise date (day/month/year) of the interview is reported, a feature that is particularly useful for our identification strategy.

Concerning smoking behavior, the SOEP asks respondents whether they smoke and, if they do, how many cigarettes and other tobacco products they smoke per day. Table A1 (in the Appendix) reports the proportion of smokers by state derived from the 2008 wave and the daily consumption of cigarettes. We observe some variation in smoking prevalence across states; while in Saarland only 20 percent report of being smokers, this proportion is as high as 32 percent in Berlin. There is less variation in smoking intensity, as the average number of cigarettes per day ranges between 13 and 18.

We also consider three indicators of social capital, two inspired by recent theoretical and empirical literature and one that was often used in the earlier literature but is less firmly theoretically grounded. Guiso *et al.* (2008, 2010) define social capital as an individual belief about the willingness of other members of the community to cooperate, and note that direct indicators like generalized trust fit well with this definition. SOEP measures trust by asking respondents to what degree they agree (using a four-point scale) with each of three statements: (a) "On the whole one can trust people"; (b) "Nowadays one can't rely on anyone"; and (c) "If one is dealing with strangers, it is better to be careful before one can trust them." Item (a) is the most similar to the question usually used to measure generalized trust that was first included in the World Values Survey and then on many other surveys; it is formulated something like "Generally speaking, would you say that most people can be trusted?" Based on item (a), then, we define our first measure of social capital, *trust*, as a dummy that takes the value of 1 if the individual fully agrees or slightly agrees with the statement, and zero otherwise. Between 53 and 72 percent of respondents reported trusting others. (See Table A1 in the Appendix.)

Our second measure of social capital is an index, denoted *trust index*, built upon the three items (a)–(c) by means of a principal component analysis. Specifically, we take the first principal component, which explains 55 percent of the overall variation in the three items and is the only component whose eigen value exceeds 1, and we rescaled the corresponding score between 0 and 1. The average value of this index, by state, reported in Table A1, ranges between 0.42 (Brandenburg and Saxony-Anhalt) and 0.52 (Hamburg). The third measure of social capital, denoted *volunteer*, is the frequency of voluntary activities. SOEP asks respondents to indicate how often they how often they take part in voluntary office participation in clubs, associations, or social services. This question refers to active and volunteer participation in generally informal social bodies. We set *volunteer* equal to 1 when individuals responded that they performed these activities at least once a month, and zero otherwise. The summary statistics reported in Table A1 show that only 13 percent of respondents performed volunteer activities at least once per month in Saxony-Anhalt and Berlin, compared to 25 percent in Baden-Wuerttemberg.

Compared to generalized trust, the frequency of volunteer activities is a more controversial measure of social capital, although it has been largely used in the literature either in this form or in a closely related formulation. (See, for instance, d'Hombres *et al.*, 2010.) One could argue that *volunteer* is an outcome of social capital rather than social capital itself; in the literature, a measure of this kind is considered "structural" social capital, while generalized trust is considered "cognitive" social capital.

Identification Strategy and the Model

We identify the effect of smoking bans on smoking prevalence and intensity before analyzing whether the magnitude of the effect varies according to level of social capital. To identify the effect of smoking bans, we exploit the fact that SOEP interviews are carried out continuously between February and October. Therefore, for each of the German states that introduced the smoking ban between February and August 2008, part of the interviews took place in the days and months just before the smoking ban was introduced, and another part in the days and months just after. Individuals who were interviewed before the ban form the control group, while individuals interviewed after ban form the treatment group. Hence, in each state, the rule of assignment to either group depends entirely on the date of the interview, which is likely orthogonal to whether a person smokes, to how much she smokes, and to all other individual characteristics. While in each state assignment to control and treatment groups is random, the probability of assignment varies across states according to the date when the smoking ban was enacted.

Table 9.2: Pre-ban and post-ban samples by state and gender.

Federal States	Males			Females		
	Pre-ban	Post-ban	Total	Pre-ban	Post-ban	Total
North-Rhine-West.	1,557	112	1,669	1,713	130	1,843
Rhineland-Palatinate	58	294	352	67	362	429
Saarland	85	6	91	104	4	108
Berlin	280	29	309	332	33	365
Brandenburg	373	20	393	411	20	431
Saxony-Anhalt	372	20	392	405	16	421
Thuringia	407	16	423	427	20	447
Total	3,132	497	3,629	3,459	585	4,044

Source: German Socio-Economic Panel (2008).

In theory we could dispose of a pre- and a post-ban sample in 2008 for 9 of the 16 states, but in practice the resulting post-ban sample has few respondents in Bremen and Mecklenburg West-Pomerania. Therefore, we focus on only seven states: North-Rhine Westphalia, Rhineland-Palatinate, Saarland, Berlin, Brandenburg, Saxony-Anhalt, and Thuringia.

Table 9.2 reports the number of observations by state and gender in the treatment (post-ban) and control (pre-ban) groups for the seven states included in the analysis. Between 5 and 10 percent of both males and females are in the treatment group, except in Rhineland-Palatinate, where the treated accounts for more than 80 percent of the sample. Table 9.3, which reports the distribution of observations according to the month of interview, shows that most of the interviews occurred between February and March, and in all states the large majority of the interviews were carried out before the beginning of the summer. In our sample there are no observations corresponding to interviews held in October.

We checked to ensure that the randomization worked as expected, that is, whether the distributions of a selected set of observable individual characteristics (age, educational level, migrant and employment status, proportion of smokers in 2006, health conditions in 2006) are balanced between the treatment and the control samples. Results reported in Table 9.4 display for each gender the conditional mean differences and the standard errors associated with the null assumption that these differences are not significantly different from zero. Conditioning variables are state dummies and two season dummies (winter and spring). State dummies are included to take into account that the process of random assignment

Table 9.3: Month of the interview by state in the German Socio-Economic Panel (2008).

	North-Rhine-West	Rhineland-Palatinate	Saarland	Berlin	Brandenburg	Saxony-Anhalt	Thuringia	Total
Feb	1,178	319	61	243	402	210	386	2,799
Mar	927	188	47	197	231	294	282	2,166
Apr	674	140	39	117	101	197	112	1,380
May	291	71	42	33	26	53	42	558
Jun	200	22	5	22	24	23	12	308
Jul	169	33	1	41	36	26	23	329
Aug	59	7	4	21	2	10	13	116
Sep	14	1	0	0	2	0	0	17
Total	3,512	781	199	674	824	813	870	7,673

Source: German Socio-Economic Panel (2008).

varies across states according to the date the smoking ban was introduced, autonomously decided by each state, and that the timing of the introduction may have depended on state-specific characteristics. For instance, it could be that states with a high prevalence of smokers or with greater attention to public health introduced the ban earlier than others did. The two conditioning season dummies are meant to control for variations over the year in smoking consumption patterns.

Results reported in Table 9.4 confirm that we do not reject the null hypothesis that the distributions of the individual characteristics of the treatment and control groups are identical. All variables are well balanced except the proportion of males who reported in 2006 (i.e., two years earlier) that they were in very good health, which is 5 percentage points higher in the treatment group. There is also marginal statistical evidence that males in the treatment group attained about 0.5 years of education less than the controls. However, what is most important is that the proportion of people who reported being smokers in 2006 is well balanced between the treatment and control groups for both genders.

The balancing of social capital indicators is reported in the lower panel of Table 9.4. Balancing is achieved among men for all social capital indicators, but it fails for both measures related to trust for women. When we investigated this issue, we found that the problem is limited to North-Rhine Westphalia; when the state is excluded, not only differences in conditional means are not significantly

Table 9.4: Balancing property: Testing the null that the distributions of the individual characteristics of the treated and control groups are identical.

	Males		Females	
	Difference	Standard Errors	Difference	Standard Errors
Smoke in 2006	0.033	(0.043)	−0.029	(0.038)
Age	−0.965	(1.470)	0.181	(1.485)
Years of education	−0.446*	(0.261)	−0.121	(0.227)
Immigrant	−0.001	(0.013)	−0.008	(0.010)
Employed	0.012	(0.044)	−0.033	(0.043)
Very good health in 2006	0.056**	(0.024)	0.015	(0.021)
Good health in 2006	−0.051	(0.046)	−0.058	(0.042)
Satisfactory health in 2006	−0.018	(0.043)	0.008	(0.042)
Poor health in 2006	0.011	(0.030)	0.031	(0.028)
Bad health in 2006	0.001	(0.016)	0.003	(0.017)
Social Capital Indicators:				
a) All states				
Trust	0.060	(0.045)	0.113***	(0.041)
Trust index	−0.002	(0.018)	0.033**	(0.015)
Volunteer	−0.037	(0.037)	0.020	(0.032)
b) North-Rhine W. excluded				
Trust	0.035	(0.060)	0.061	(0.054)
Trust index	0.006	(0.024)	0.031	(0.020)
Volunteer	0.005	(0.043)	0.001	(0.040)

Note: The table displays (i) the conditional mean differences for the variables reported in the first column between the treated and control groups (ii) the standard errors associated with the null hypothesis that the mean differences are not significantly different from zero. Conditioning variables are state dummies and winter and spring dummies. Robust standard errors in parenthesis. $^*p < 0.1$, $^{**}p < 0.05$, $^{***}p < 0.01$.
Source: German Socio-Economic Panel (2006 and 2008).

different from zero, a fact that may depend only on the reduced sample size, but they are generally smaller.

On this conditional randomized framework we fit a simple-difference model defined as

$$Y_{is1} = \alpha_0 + \alpha_1 ban_{is1} + \beta Y_{is0} + X_{is}\gamma + \varepsilon_{is} \tag{9.1}$$

where Y_{is1} and Y_{is0} are the outcome variables in 2008 and 2006, respectively. We consider two complementary outcomes: Whether individual i residing in state s

in 2008 reports being a smoker and the number of cigarettes individual i smoked per day, measured in number of half-packs (five cigarettes). The treatment variable ban_{is1} is a dummy that takes the value of 1 if individual i residing in state s in 2008 was interviewed after the introduction of the smoking ban and zero otherwise. Controls included in the vector X_{is} are individual health conditions in 2006 (i.e., two years earlier), age, a second-order polynomial of years of schooling, as well as state dummies and two season dummies (winter and spring), which are required in order to account for the variation by state in the randomization process. Finally, ε_{is} is the error term. The parameter of interest is α_1, which captures the effect of the introduction of the smoking ban on the considered outcome.

Inclusion of the lagged outcome in model (9.1) renders model (9.1) a value-added model that evaluates how the introduction of the smoking ban affected individuals' changes in smoking status and the number of cigarettes smoked.[42] Given that Y_{is0} is orthogonal to ban_{is1}, its inclusion will not affect the point estimate of α_1. Rather, it improves the precision of our estimates, as it increases the model's goodness of fit.

The identification strategy that we use to estimate α_1 is different from the one adopted in Anger et al. (2010). In our case, the effect of the smoking ban on smoking behavior is identified because in 2008, in 7 of the 16 German states, some individuals were subject to the smoking ban at the time of the interview, while others were still free to smoke in public spaces. The key condition to obtain unbiased estimates of α_1 is that, in each state, the assignment to the treatment and control groups is random. Angers et al. (2011) consider all 16 states and rely on four waves of SOEP (2002, 2004, 2006, and 2008), but their identification strategy requires stronger assumptions. They estimate a difference-in-differences model that assumes a "common trend,"[43] but the validity of the common trend assumption is crucial if an unbiased estimate of α_1 is to be obtained. Especially in this context, where the effect of the smoking ban appears to be small and easily hidden or confounded by even small model misspecifications, any deviation from the "common trend" could lead to wrong conclusions.

---

[42]Alternatively, model (9.1) can be thought of as a difference-in-differences model. (See, e.g., Hanusheck and Woessman, 2006.)

[43]Angers et al. (2011) assume that, in the absence of smoking bans, both the treatment group and the control group would have experienced the same trend in smoking prevalence and intensity.

To determine how social capital modifies the effect of the smoking ban, we consider an extension of model (9.1):

$$Y_{is1} = \alpha_0 + \alpha_1 ban_{is1} + \alpha_2 ban_{is1} * SC_{is1} + \alpha_3 SC_{is1} + \beta Y_{is0} + X_{is}\gamma + \mu_s + \varepsilon_{is}$$
(9.2)

in which the interaction between individual social capital SC_{is1} and ban_{is1} is added. The marginal effect of the smoking ban is given by $\alpha_1 + \alpha_2 SC_{is1}$, which is larger for individuals who are rich in social capital if both α_1 and α_2 are negative. As is widely recognized elsewhere (Durlauf and Fafchamps, 2005; Rocco and Fumagalli in this book), individual social capital is likely to be correlated with individual preferences and unobservable traits. One reason for this correlation is that social capital, along with time and risk preferences, is transmitted by parents. As parents tend to protect their children, more risk-averse parents likely transmit more pessimistic beliefs about the average willingness of the population to cooperate than do less risk-averse parents (Guiso et al., 2008). However, as is shown in the Appendix, because the assignment to the treatment and control groups is random, the coefficient α_2, which captures the influence of social capital on the ban's effectiveness, will be unbiased in spite of the endogeneity of SC_{is1}.[44]

Results

Table 9.5 reports our baseline results about the effect of the smoking ban on smoking prevalence. When we estimated model (9.1) by gender on the entire sample (columns 1 and 2) we find a moderate and marginally significant effect of the smoking ban only on males. The probability of smoking is about 4 percent lower among males. No significant effect is seen among females, — and the sign of the point estimate is even opposite to what we expected. These results are in line with Anger et al. (2011). The same pattern by gender arises when we limit our attention to males and females who reported of being smokers in 2006. The corresponding estimates are displayed in columns (3) and (4). We find that the introduction of the ban reduced significantly the probability of smoking in 2008 by a noteworthy 13 percent among male former smokers and that it had no effect on female former smokers.

---

[44]Of course, the estimate of parameter α_3 will be biased.

Table 9.5: Effect of smoking ban on smoking prevalence.

	(1)	(2)	(3)	(4)	(5)
	All		Former Smokers		
	Males	Females	Males	Females	Males by Age
Smoking ban	−0.042*	0.0286	−0.136***	0.0261	−0.0387*
	(0.023)	(0.022)	(0.049)	(0.065)	(0.023)
Smoking ban interacted with a young dummy					−0.136
					(0.091)
Young dummy					0.0050
					(0.047)
Observations	3,249	3,655	1,059	998	3,249
R-squared	0.660	0.666	0.020	0.014	0.660

Note: Linear probability model. The dependent variable is a dummy variable taking the value 1 if the individual reports to be a smoker, 0 otherwise. All regressions include: lagged smoke, age, years of education, squared years of education, lagged health condition dummies, state dummies, winter and spring dummies. The young dummy (column 5) takes the value 1 if the individual is less than 21 year-old, 0 otherwise. Robust standard errors in parenthesis. $^*p < 0.$, $^{**}p < 0.05$, $^{***}p < 0.01$.
Source: German Socio-Economic Panel (2006 and 2008).

In Table 9.6, columns 1 and 2, we report the effect of the smoking ban on the consumption of cigarettes per day. As Jones *et al.* (2011) note, since people tend to report the number of cigarettes they smoke in multiples of five, we use the number of half-packs smoked per day instead of the number of cigarettes smoked per day as the dependent variable. Equation (9.1) is estimated using a Poisson model, and the structural parameters are reported. The marginal effect of the introduction of the ban is significant only for males, pointing to a reduction of 0.6 half-packs per day,[45] or about three cigarettes per day. The effect is negative but not statistically significant for females.

Since young people are more likely than others to attend public places (Anger *et al.*, 2011),[46] we test whether there is any differential effect of the smoking ban in terms of smoking prevalence and intensity among males younger than 21. In

---

[45]Marginal effects are roughly three times larger than the structural parameters of the Poisson model reported in Table 9.6.
[46]In addition, it might be easier for them to comply with the smoking ban, as their degree of addiction to tobacco is likely to be lower compared to that of older smokers.

Table 9.6: Effect of smoking ban on smoking intensity of former smokers.

	(1) Males	(2) Females	(3) Males by Age
Smoking ban	−0.211**	−0.105	−0.208**
	(0.084)	(0.10)	(0.083)
Smoking ban interacted with a young dummy			−0.309
			(0.426)
Young dummy			−0.161
			(0.133)
Observations	947	967	947

Note: Poisson model. The dependent variable is the number of half packs (5 cigarettes) smoked every day. All specifications include: lagged number of half packs smoked, age, years of education, squared years of education, lagged health condition dummies, state dummies, winter and spring dummies. The young dummy (column 5) takes the value 1 if the individual is less than 21 year-old, 0 otherwise. Sample limited to the former smokers. Robust standard errors in parenthesis. $*p < 0.1$, $**p < 0.05$, $***p < 0.01$.
Source: German Socio-Economic Panel (2006 and 2008).

both column 5 of Table 9.5 and column 3 of Table 9.6, the sign of the interaction is negative but not statistically significant.

Finally, we estimate the models for smoking prevalence and intensity for males using all German states, including the states that introduced the ban before February 2008. For these states all respondents are in the treatment group. As state dummies have been introduced, these states will not contribute to the identification of the ban effect. Moreover, being the common support requirement violated, the effect of the treatment conditional to residing in one of these states can be identified only by means of the functional form assumed in the model. In our case, estimates are slightly smaller, as Table A3 in the Appendix shows, but qualitative results for all of Germany roughly confirm those obtained from the baseline specification.

Overall, we find that smoking bans had a moderate effect on males but no effect on females and that, among smokers, the likelihood that they continued to smoke after the ban fell by 13 percent and the average number of cigarettes smoked per day decreased by two or three.

Next, we examine whether the effect of smoking bans is stronger for individuals who are richer in social capital by investigating how three indicators of social capital — generalized trust, an index of trust, and the frequency of volunteer activities — mediate the effect of the smoking ban. Given that the effect of the smoking bans is more evident among men, we discuss in detail results for this sub-group only.

Tables 9.7 and 9.8 report estimates of model (2) for all men (smokers and non-smokers) interviewed in 2008 and for the subset of male former smokers. Table 9.7 shows that individual social capital strengthens the effect of the smoking bans in terms of smoking prevalence. In particular, looking at column 1, bans reduce smoking prevalence by 6 percent among men who report a high level of generalized trust (i.e., *trust* = 1), while there is no effect among men who report a low level of trust (i.e., *trust* = 0). Less clear results are found when the *trust index* is considered (column 2); while there is no significant differential effect in the ban effect that is due to the level of *trust index*, the marginal effect of the smoking ban given by $\alpha_1 + \alpha_2 SC_{is1}$ is significantly different from zero, indicating that the probability that a man smokes is reduced by 11 percent when *trust index* = 1, while the effect is practically zero when *trust index* = 0. Little evidence of differential effects is found when the variable *volunteer* is used (column 3). In this case, the marginal effect of the ban amounts to a reduction in smoking prevalence of 7 percent among men who perform volunteer activities, compared to a non-significant 3 percent reduction among men who are less involved in these activities. Qualitatively similar results are obtained when we focus on the subset of male former smokers (columns 4–6), where point estimates are larger but their precision is generally smaller, probably because of the limited sample size.

For smoking intensity (Table 9.8), we find that the two measures of social capital related to trust significantly influence the effect of the smoking ban on the number of half packs smoked per day whether we consider the entire sample (the number of half-packs smoked per day is set to zero for non-smokers) or the restricted sample of male former smokers. On the other hand, when social capital is measured by participation in voluntary activities, we cannot conclude that social capital mediates the effect of the smoking ban, thus confirming our previous findings on smoking prevalence.[47]

---

[47]For completeness, we also estimated model (9.2) on the sample of women, in spite of the absence of any significant effect of the smoking ban for this group and although the distribution of social capital between the treatment and control groups was not identical for females. We obtained results qualitatively similar to those for men, although they were statistically significant only for smoking intensity. This is the case both when North-Rhine Westphalia, the state responsible for unbalancing, is included and when it is not. Results are available upon request.

Table 9.7: Social capital and smoking ban on smoking prevalence of males.

	(1)	(2)	(3)	(4)	(5)	(6)
	All			Former Smokers		
Smoking ban	−0.003	0.014	−0.035	−0.080	−0.103	−0.122**
	(0.029)	(0.044)	(0.025)	(0.060)	(0.082)	(0.050)
Smoking ban interacted with *trust*	−0.064** (0.030)			−0.094 (0.066)		
Trust	0.021* (0.011)			0.021 (0.023)		
Smoking ban interacted with *trust index*		−0.124 (0.081)			−0.084 (0.153)	
Trust index		0.061** (0.030)			0.070 (0.066)	
Smoking ban interacted with *volunteer*			−0.036 (0.031)			−0.108 (0.109)
Volunteer			0.001 (0.012)			0.035 (0.030)
Observations	3,242	3,237	3,244	1,057	1,056	1,057
R-squared	0.660	0.660	0.660	0.022	0.020	0.021
$\alpha_1 + \alpha_2 SC_{is1}$	−0.0674***	−0.110**	−0.0709**	−0.174***	−0.187*	−0.230**
	(0.026)	(0.049)	(0.021)	(0.057)	(0.099)	(0.110)

Note: See Table 9.6. *Trust* is a variable taking the value 1 if the individual reports to fully or slightly agree with the statement that "on the whole, one can trust people", 0 otherwise. The *trust index* is a based on the following questions: (1) "On the whole one can trust people"; (2) "Nowadays one can't rely on anyone"; (3) "If one is dealing with strangers, it is better to be careful before one can trust them". A principal component analysis was used to combine the three measures into a single variable. *Volunteer* is a variable taking the value one if the individuals reports to take part in honorary office participation in clubs, associations or social services at least once per month, 0 otherwise. The linear combination of the coefficient of ban and of the coefficient associated to the interaction between ban and each social capital indicator as well as its associated standard errors are reported in the last row of the table.

Table 9.8: Social capital and smoking ban on smoking intensity. Dependent variable: Number of half packs.

	(1)	(2)	(3)	(4)	(5)	(6)
	All			Former Smokers		
Smoking ban	0.020	0.488**	−0.247*	−0.048	0.080	−0.196**
	(0.144)	(0.200)	(0.139)	(0.100)	(0.132)	(0.086)
Smoking ban interacted with trust	−0.487*** (0.165)			−0.267*** (0.101)		
Trust	−0.044 (0.070)			0.006 (0.039)		
Smoking ban interacted with trust index		−1.729*** (0.439)			−0.667*** (0.259)	
Trust index		0.233 (0.255)			0.041 (0.124)	
Smoking ban interacted with volunteer			−0.048 (0.233)			−0.115 (0.153)
Volunteer			−0.212** (0.076)			−0.043 (0.053)
Observations	3,113	3,108	3,115	945	944	945
$\alpha_1 + \alpha_2 SC_{is1}$	−0.467***	−1.240***	−0.295	−0.315***	−0.587***	−0.311**
	(0.163)	(0.309)	(0.234)	(0.094)	(0.175)	(0.157)

Note: See Table 9.6. Trust is a variable taking the value 1 if the individual reports to fully or slightly agree with the statement that "on the whole, one can trust people," 0 otherwise. The trust index is a based on the following questions: (1) "On the whole one can trust people"; (2) "Nowadays one can't rely on anyone"; (3) "If one is dealing with strangers, it is better to be careful before one can trust them." A principal component analysis was used to combine the 3 measures into a single variable. Volunteer is a variable taking the value one if the individuals reports to take part in honorary office participation in clubs, associations or social services at least once per month, 0 otherwise. The linear combination of the coefficient of ban and of the coefficient associated to the interaction between ban and each social capital indicator as well as its associated standard errors are reported in the last row of the table.

More specifically, we find that, among male former smokers, the effect of the smoking ban conditional on *trust* = 1 is equivalent to a reduction of about a half pack (i.e., 5 cigarettes per day), compared to an effect that is not significantly different from zero when we condition to *trust* = 0 (column 4). When the social capital mediator adopted is the *trust index*, we find that the effect of the smoking ban is a reduction of 1.5 half packs per day among men with the highest level of social capital (*trust index* = 1) and not significant (and actually with the sign reversed) among those with the lowest level of social capital (*trust index* = 0). Since the trust index averages about 0.4, the marginal effect of the ban evaluated at the average of the trust index is a reduction of about 0.6 half packs per day (column 5).

We report estimates for the entire sample of men (columns 1–3) including male non-smokers in 2006, in order to improve comparability between Tables 9.7 and 9.8. Results from the sample of male former smokers and the entire sample are absolutely in line. Although point estimates are much larger in the latter, marginal effects are similar.[48]

Summary and Concluding Remarks

To the best of our knowledge, this is the first study to investigate the possibility that one of the mechanisms proposed in the literature explains the negative effect of social capital on smoking prevalence and intensity. Moreover, for the first time in the literature on social capital and health, this study uses a quasi-experimental setting and program evaluation techniques.

The goal of this chapter has been to determine whether the effect of smoking bans introduced in Germany between 2007 and 2008 is stronger for individuals who are rich in social capital than for those who are not. According to the literature, enforcement of and compliance with anti-smoking regulations should be stronger among communities with higher levels of social capital and among more socially oriented individuals. Our empirical results confirm this prediction, at least for males. Specifically, the effect of the bans in terms of both smoking prevalence and smoking intensity is nil among men with low levels of social capital, while it is comparatively strong among more trusting and socially inclined men.

---

[48]For instance, the marginal effect conditional to *trust* = 1 is a reduction in cigarettes consumption of 0.45 half packs per day, and the one conditional to *trust index* = 1 is a reduction of 1.2 half packs per day.

Given the estimation strategy adopted, the effects of the smoking ban we found must be considered short-run effects. It is not clear *a priori* whether such effects will strengthen or weaken as time passes and smoking bans become more firmly established. Predictions are further complicated by the decision of the Federal Constitutional Court to allow small bars to become "smoking pubs," a rule that may have reduced the overall effectiveness of the smoking bans. Nevertheless, we believe that looking at short-run effects is appropriate in observing and analyzing the mediating role of social capital since factors like peer effects, habit, additional regulation changes, and variations in cigarette prices could alter and confound the picture.

There are three potential concerns about the current analysis that are worth discussing. First, the introduction of smoking bans is an event expected and perfectly anticipated. Some states enforced the ban only some months after its introduction in order to allow people to become familiar with the new rules, so it is possible that smoking behavior changed before the date the ban was enacted. For instance, people could have stopped smoking in public places before the ban was enforced or, conversely, people could have smoked more, anticipating the coming restriction. If either of these conditions was the case, our identification strategy could either understate or overstate the effect of the ban. To address this possibility, we looked at smoking prevalence before and after "placebo" dates that precede the true introduction dates and found no significant effect of the enforcement in any of the cases.

Second, for some states, such as Saarland, Brandenburg, Saxony-Anhalt, and Thuringia, the treatment sample is small, which could impact the reliability of our estimates. We reproduced our key estimates for the sample using only North-Rhine Westphalia, Rhineland-Palatinate, and Berlin and found similar point estimates with only a minor loss of precision. Therefore, we conclude that the problem of small sample size is likely unimportant.

Third, and perhaps most problematic, is whether the date of the interview is really orthogonal to individual characteristics. This claim is supported by the balancing tests we performed, but the relatively small sample used could have hidden an underlying structural correlation behind the scarce precision of the estimates. Suppose, for instance, that people interviewed later are those who were difficult to find at their addresses. These people could be the busiest, those who work farthest from their place of residence, or immigrants whose place of residence is more difficult to determine. Reversing this argument, older people and retired people could be interviewed earlier because they are more easily found at their addresses. If this was the case, there could be a correlation between the assignment to the treatment group and some individual characteristics. We cannot entirely exclude this possibility, but the balancing tests are reassuring in this respect since they reveal small differences in the employment rate and immigrant status between the treatment group and the control group, especially so for males. To further support the case for random assignment between treatment and control group we tested whether the proportion of civil servants differs among the two groups. The reason is that civil servants typically work closer to home than do people employed in other occupations. If the respondents interviewed earlier are those who are more likely to work near their residence (and therefore, easier for SOEP interviewers to find at their addresses), we should observe a higher proportion of civil servants among the control group and a lower proportion among the treatment group. We checked whether the proportion of civil servants in the treatment group and the control group is balanced, conditional to the control variables included in models (9.1) and (9.2), and found no evidence of unbalancing for either gender. These results reinforce the plausibility of our claim that the date of interview can be considered a random event.

Appendix A

In this Appendix, we show that the parameter α_2 of model (9.2), estimated by means of OLS, correctly identifies the component of the smoking ban effect depending on individual social capital.

Given X and μ_s and the level of individual social capital $SC_{is1} = k$, we compute the following conditional expectation for $ban_{is1} = 1$ and $ban_{is1} = 0$, respectively:

$$E(Y_{is1}|ban_{is1} = 1, SC_{is1} = k, X, \mu_s)$$
$$= \alpha_0 + \alpha_1 + \alpha_2 k + \alpha_3 k + X\beta + \mu_s + E(\varepsilon_{is}|ban_{is1} = 1, SC_{is1} = k, X, \mu_s)$$
$$E(Y_{is1}|ban_{is1} = 0, SC_{is1} = k, X, \mu_s)$$
$$= \alpha_0 + \alpha_3 k + X\beta + \mu_s + E(\varepsilon_{is}|ban_{is1} = 0, SC_{is1} = k, X, \mu_s)$$

Being $E(\varepsilon_{is}|ban_{is1} = 1, SC_{is1} = k, X, \mu_s) = E(\varepsilon_{is}|ban_{is1} = 0, SC_{is1} = k, X, \mu_s)$ due to the conditional randomness of the treatment variable, the effect of the smoking ban when individual level of social capital is k is given by:

$$E(Y_{is1}|ban_{is1} = 1, SC_{is1} = k, X, \mu_s) - E(Y_{is1}|ban_{is1} = 0, SC_{is1} = k, X, \mu_s)$$
$$= \alpha_1 + \alpha_2 k$$

Appendix B

Table A1: Smoking prevalence and intensity — Summary statistics.

State	Proportion of Smokers (%)	No. of Cigarettes Per Day Among Smokers
North-Rhine-Westphalia	29.21	16.0
Rhineland-Palatinate	26.89	16.9
Saarland	21.61	17.7
Berlin	32.20	14.5
Brandenburg	27.43	14.1
Saxony-Anhalt	30.75	13.7
Thuringia	25.06	13.0
Schleswig-Holstein	25.14	15.8
Hamburg	26.77	13.5
Lower Saxony	27.22	15.9
Bremen	26.52	15.0
Hessen	27.92	14.3
Baden-Wurttemberg	22.87	15.0
Bavaria	26.54	14.9
Mecklenburg West -Pomerania	31.17	15.2
Saxony	23.27	12.6

Source: 2008 German Socio-Economic Panel.

Table A2: Measures of social capital — Summary statistics.

Federal State	Proportion Individuals Who Report to Trust Others	Average Generalized Trust Index	Proportion of Individuals Who Report to Perform Volunteer Activities at Least Once a Month
North-Rhine-Westphalia	62.09	0.46	17.67
Rhineland-Palatinate	60.85	0.46	18.69
Saarland	60.91	0.44	21.72
Berlin	60.48	0.48	12.91
Brandenburg	54.98	0.42	14.46
Saxony-Anhalt	53.15	0.42	12.84
Thuringia	56.90	0.44	16.13
Schleswig-Holstein	71.79	0.51	15.19
Hamburg	68.91	0.52	19.85
Lower Saxony	64.19	0.47	22.64
Bremen	62.88	0.49	18.18
Hessen	64.83	0.47	20.93
Baden-Wurttemberg	67.91	0.49	25.39
Bavaria	62.92	0.47	21.95
Mecklenburg West-Pomerania	55.58	0.44	18.37
Saxony	56.35	0.44	13.93

Source: 2008 German Socio-Economic Panel; Column 2 displays the proportion of individuals who report to fully or slightly agree with the statement that "on the whole, one can trust people." Column 3 is a trust index based on the three following questions: (1) "On the whole one can trust people"; (2) "Nowadays one can't rely on anyone"; (3) "If one is dealing with strangers, it is better to be careful before one can trust them." A principal component analysis was used to combine the 3 measures into a single variable. The trust index ranges between 0 and 1. The last column is the proportion of individuals who report to take part in honorary office participation in clubs, associations or social services at least once per month.

Table A3: Effect of the smoking ban on smoking prevalence and intensity in all 16 German states.

	(1) Smoking Males	(2) Prevalence Males, Former Smokers	(3) Smoking Intensity Males
Smoking ban	−0.030	−0.104**	−0.185**
	(0.021)	(0.048)	(0.083)
Observations	7,616	2,374	2,143
R-squared	0.652	0.021	

Note: See Table 9.5 for columns (1) and (2) and Table 9.6 for column (3).

References

Anger, S., Kvasnicka, M. and Siedlera, T. 2011. One last puff? Public smoking bans and smoking behavior. *Journal of Health Economics*, 30: 591–601.

Brown, T. T., Colla, C. H. and Scheffler, R. M. 2011. Does community-level social capital affect smoking behavior? An instrumental variables approach. Mimeo.

Buonanno , P. and Ranzani, M. 2012. Thank you for not smoking: Evidence from the Italian smoking ban. *Health Policy*, 109(2): 192–199.

d'Hombres, B., Rocco, L., Suhrcke, M. and McKee, M. 2010. Does social capital determine health? Evidence from eight transition countries. *Health Economics*, 19(1): 56–74.

Durlauf, S. N. and Fafchamps, M. 2005. Social capital. In *Handbook of Economic Growth*, eds. Aghion, P. and Durlauf, S.N., Elsevier, pp. 1639–1699.

Folland, S. 2006. Value of life and behavior toward health risks: An interpretation of social capital. *Health Economics*, 15: 159–171.

Folland, S., Islam, K. and Oddvar, K. 2011. The social capital and health hypothesis: A theory and new empirics featuring the Norwegian HUNT data. Mimeo.

Göhlmann, S. and Schmidt, C. M. 2008. Smoking in Germany: Stylized facts, behavioral models, and health policy. Ruhr Economic Papers No. 64.

Guiso, L., Sapienza, P. and Zingales, L. 2010. Civic capital as the missing link. National Bureau of Economic Research Working Paper No. 15845.

Guiso, L., Sapienza, P. and Zingales, L. 2008. Alfred Marshall Lecture: Social capital as good culture. *Journal of the European Economic Association*, 6(2–3): 295–320.

Hanushek, E. A. and Wossmann, L. 2006. Does educational tracking affect performance and inequality? Differences-in-differences evidence across countries. *The Economic Journal*, 116: C63–C76.

Jones, A. M., Laporte, A., Rice, N. and Zucchelli, E. 2011. A model of the impact of smoking bans on smoking with evidence from bans in England and Scotland. HEDG WP 5/11.

Kvasnicka, M. 2010. Public smoking bans, youth access laws, and cigarette sales at vending machines. Ruhr Economic Papers No. 173.

Li, S. and Delva, J. 2011. Does gender moderate associations between social capital and smoking? An Asian American study. *Health Behavior and Public Health*, 1(1): 41–49.

Li, S. and Delva, J. 2012. Social capital and smoking among Asian American men: An exploratory study. *American Journal of Public Health*, 102(2): S212–S221.

Lindström, M. 2003. Social capital and the miniaturization of community among daily and intermittent smokers: A population-based study. *Preventive Medicine*, 36(2): 177–184.

Lindström, M. 2008. Social capital and health-related behaviors. In *Social Capital and Health*, eds. Kawachi, I., Subramanian, S. V. and Kim, D., New York: Springer, pp. 215–238.

Lindström, M. 2009. Social capital, political trust and daily smoking and smoking cessation: A population-based study in southern Sweden. *Public Health*, 123(7): 496–501.

Lundborg P. 2005. Social capital and substance use among Swedish adolescents — An explorative study. *Social Science & Medicine*, 61(6): 1151–1158.

Origo, F. and Lucifora, C. 2010. The effect of comprehensive smoking bans in European workplace. IZA DP. 5290.

Rocco, L. and Fumagalli, E. 2014. The emprics of social capital and health. *In The Economics of Social Capital and Health: A Conceptual and Empirical Roadmap*, eds. Folland, S. and Rocco, L. Singapore: World Scientific.

Takakura, M. 2011. Does social trust at school affect students' smoking and drinking behavior in Japan? *Social Science and Medicine*, 72: 299–306.

Tampubolon, G., Subramanian, S. V. and Kawachi, I. 2011. Neighbourhood social capital and individual self-rated health in Wales. *Health Economics*, 22(1): 14–21.

Todd, P. E. and Wolpin, K. I. 2003. On the specification and estimation of the production function for cognitive achievement. *The Economic Journal*, 113(485): F3–F33.

Wagner, G. G., Frick, F. R. and Schupp, J. 2007. The German Socio-Economic Panel Study (SOEP) — Scope, evolution and enhancements. *Schmollers Jahrbuch* 127(1): 139–169.

Chapter 10

Policy Implications

Eline Aas

Introduction

The previous chapters reviewed the literature on the effect of social capital on health considering both theoretical and empirical approaches, including the effects of individual social capital and community social capital on health. Empirical findings have shown an effect of social capital on health for several dimensions of social capital, such as marital status, working status, number of friends, religious participation, community trust, and voting participation. The focus of this chapter is the policy implications that could be derived from the findings. Accordingly, we discuss for each finding or group of findings policies the government could take to improve health through increased investments in social capital.

Definitions related to the multi-faceted concept of social capital, including which types of social structures can be defined as social capital and how social capital can be measured in empirical studies, are continuously under revision and development in search of the most explicit and concise definitions. A concise definition of social capital is a prerequisite to outlining policy implications. As the development of measurements of social capital is ongoing, framing policy could be challenging.

Given a causal relationship between social capital and health, policies that could motivate individuals or communities to invest in health are much needed. Hence, to address policies, we must understand the mechanisms that *create* social capital (Figure 10.1). The subsection 'Theoretical Implications' presents the theoretical implications for policy based on the theory of investment in social capital and the transmission of social capital over generations. As there are almost no studies of the effect of policy interventions on investment in social capital, most of

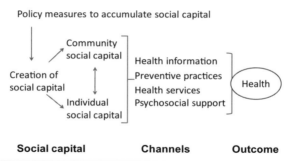

Figure 10.1: The connection between creation/investments in social capital and pathways between social capital and health (expansion of Scheffler et al., 2008).

the examples are suggestions that need to be evaluated in future research. The subsection 'Empirical Findings and Policy Implications' presents specific policy implications based on findings in the empirical literature on the effect of social capital on health outcomes and channels for health. New types of networks, such as social networks on the internet, are discussed in 'New Types of Networks', and concluding remarks are given in the 'Summary and Concluding Remarks'.

Theoretical Implications

The policy implications derived from the theoretical literature on how social capital is created define the baseline for the discussion in this section. Policies to increase individual social capital, how community social capital could be increased, and how interactions between individual and community social capital could have implications for policy are discussed.

Individual social capital

Factors that affect the individual's investments in social capital must be emphasized when designing relevant policies for the creation of social capital. As social capital is an important factor in progress in several areas in addition to health, sustaining social capital is important from the governmental, individual, and institutional/group points of view.

Based on the framework from Gleaser *et al.* (2002) and Grossman (1972), the investment decision is affected by factors like the aggregate stock of social capital in the community, each individual's market and non-market return from the community stock of social capital, the depreciation rate, the opportunity cost of time (wage rate), mobility, and the discount factor, and the investment in social capital is restricted by the budget constraint that reflects the costs of investing. Based on the model, the comparative statics state that accumulation in individual social capital (a) declines with mobility, the opportunity cost of time, the rate of depreciation, the rate of social capital depreciation resulting from relocation, and age, and (b) increases with the discount factor, occupational return to social skills and in communities with more social capital (Gleaser et al., 2002).

The model presented in Gleaser et al. (2002) is a general framework that is not directly related to health but has been adapted to the literature on social capital on health in several papers (Islam et al., 2006; Scheffler, 2007).

Based on the predictions in the model, individuals accumulate social capital when the private incentives for accumulations are high. In summary, social capital tends to be accumulated among young people living in a stable community characterized by a high stock of social capital, low mobility, and a high degree of homeownership, and among those with an occupation with a high return to social skills. One would expect that the stock of health is high for these people as well.

Policy should be designed to accumulate social capital in order to ensure social inclusion, as social inclusion is a key component of high returns in several arenas, including health (e.g., Scheffler and Brown, 2008). Standard policies that could be considered are financial incentives and taxations, regulations (privileges), campaigns at the community and national level, and facilitating organizations and services.

The predictions from the models indicate a close relationship between human capital and social capital, as investment in these two types of capital accumulates when skills have high returns. However, unlike policies for investments in human capital, where the government has a distinct position in framing policy with regard to both education and employment, the government has a less distinct position in framing policy with regard to investment in social capital. Even though the government's power to influence is less distinct on the individual level, it could still be strong on the aggregate level. Interventions at the aggregate level will be discussed in the next section.

The most relevant policies for stimulating investments in social capital in order to achieve improved health could be financial incentives and facilitating access to social networks. When designing policy, it is also important to recognize that the needs of seemingly equal individuals may differ and that needs change over time.

The following are several examples of financial-incentive policies: To encourage increased investments in social capital on the individual level, financial incentives could be directed at organizations and at individuals. For instance, organizations could receive subsidies if they are willing to extend the number of groups in a community, such as AA groups and support groups for people living with cancer and cardiovascular diseases. Doing so would reduce the physical distance to a network, which Glaeser *et al.* (2002) finds has a positive effect on investment in social capital, as reduction of physical distance to such groups reduces the cost of investing in social capital. Such a measure could be an important tool in maintaining accumulation of social capital for individuals who experience high costs of investing in social capital and/or those who would gain significant health benefits through increased social capital. Women who recently gave birth and the elderly are examples of two broad groups that might have both high costs and potential health benefits of investing in social capital.

For parents, providing free access to a clinic for newborns could be a way to observe the health of the child and give the parents the opportunity to join other parents with children of the same age and living in the same area. Such groups might result in an accumulation of social capital over time for the parents as well as the child(ren). Through these networks shared information could lead to positive health gains. Such policy measures are widely used in several countries, including the UK, Sweden, and Norway.

Deprivation of health care increases with age as the need for health care increases, so there is a potential health gain in ensuring accumulation of social capital as long as possible in order to compensate for or at least mitigate the deprivation of health care. Financial incentives such as partial or full subsidies for membership fees in social organizations, could be applied to motivate investments in social capital. Using a direct subsidy might be more effective than, say, a tax deduction, as transaction costs will be lower. Another alternative is to subsidize costs related to social activities like transportation by allocating free taxi rides.

The family is an important source of social capital, so financial incentives to lighten the burden for relatives of the elderly, such as days off of work to care for parents, could substitute for other types of social networks. Fevang *et al.* (2012) studied the labor supply among relatives of lone parents and found that the labor supply is significantly reduced during the terminal stages of lone parents' lives and, for some people, also after the parent's death. As labor supply is correlated with the relative's health state, more flexible welfare arrangements would reduce the burden and may secure the family network. Such a policy measure could also be an important measure for other groups with high costs of investing in social capital, such as children and the disabled.

Mobility is predicted to have a negative effect on the accumulation of social capital, so securing stable living conditions by using financial incentives to lighten the burden of becoming a homeowner could help in the accumulation of social capital. Policies like zero tax on savings earmarked for investments in homes and tax deductions for interest on mortgages would help to grow the number of homeowners (Norwegian Ministry of Finance, 2011)

Many of these policies already exist in various countries. Future research should determine which new policies are the most effective by studying which result in an accumulation of social capital and, consequently, an effect on health, and which do not.

Community social capital

Community social capital could be defined as the sum of, the distribution of, or the average of social capital in a community, such as the proportion of civic engagement (or civic capital) and trust. A high level of social capital in a community is an important factor in improving health, as Putnam (1993) first showed. The purpose of the policies is to create a trusting and stable community that stimulates social interactions by reducing transaction costs. As trust and reciprocity are dynamic characteristics that require time to develop, one overall important policy implication might be that it is important for government to provide stable and predictable policies.

In a theoretical framework developed and used by Tabellini (2008), Guiso et al. (2004, 2008) and Aghion et al. (2008) made a clear distinction between social capital and physical and human capital that represented a change from the models discussed earlier. In this framework, unlike human and physical capital, social capital has the potential to accumulate over time. In these models, social capital is defined through civic capital and/or trust, and the investments differ from human capital because of social interactions. In the model presented in Tabellini (2008), values and attitudes are transferred from parents to children and are based on traditional economic assumptions. Since the parents make a rational decision about which values to transfer to their children, the children's welfare is defined in terms of the parent's values. There is a complementary relationship between values and behavior, as strengthened values or the scope of cooperation ease the transmission of values. From generation to generation, these transmissions are amplified.

Guiso *et al.* (2008) present an overlapping-generation model in which, similar to Tabellini (2008), social capital, such as trust, is transferred between generations. Here, the parents' priors are explicitly defined and transmitted to their children. As children and parents value the past and the future differently, parents tend to transmit over-conservative priors in order to reduce risk that their children are exploited by other people in their future life.

The models presented by Tabellini (2008), Guiso *et al.* (2004, 2008) and Aghion *et al.* (2008) all explain the transmission of values like trust within families, but they could also be applied to communities, even though community ties may not be as strong as family ties. Based on the theoretical models, then, which policies could be applied to increase community social capital? Here are some suggestions:

Financial incentives: Financial incentives could be used to motivate a high degree of social interaction in a community by encouraging the establishment of organizations, subsidizing organizations, or reducing the value-added tax for voluntary organizations, sports organizations, and support groups.

Regulations: To reduce crime rates and increase safety in local communities, regulations could be used to facilitate the establishment of community organizations. In addition, since health care services constitute a combination of services that could be offered at different governmental levels and could have very different characteristics, regulations could ease the logistics for individuals through local support groups to ensure optimal treatment, especially for individuals with large and complex needs. A regulation that ensures access to support groups that assist individuals in need could improve their health through a formal network.

Regulations could also be used to change social benefits, such as requiring employers to accept their employees' work in voluntary and civic activities, rather than punishing it with reduced pay or leave time. For example, regulations could be used along with financial compensation to either the employer or the employee to support participation in a jury, efforts in civil preparedness, the Red Cross, or other caring groups.

The strong relationship between mistrust and the level of regulation is discussed in Aghion *et al.* (2008). Regulations must be able to adjust for externalities in communities with low levels of civic capital, such as those with high degrees of tax evasion. Guiso *et al.* (2010) also suggested that education is an important tool with which to increase civic engagement. In a publicly funded school system, children are less dependent on transmission of values and beliefs from their parents because they can accumulate values and beliefs during their education. Therefore, ensuring the right to public education could increase civic engagement. Civic capital in a community is a public good that helps everyone accumulate gains.

Campaigns: Campaigns could be used to increase the flow of knowledge and encourage social interaction, voting, and civic engagements. For instance, campaigns could be used to inform a community about positive trends in the crime rate. Knowing that one's neighborhood is safe would reduce the barriers to social interaction as trust increases. Campaigns could also be used to inform communities about regulations designed to enhance social capital.

One important effect of social capital is the access that individuals get to information through the network. The healthcare sector is characterized by asymmetric information between, for instance, the doctor and the patient, so a larger network could reduce the asymmetry, as the network could share information with patients on medications, diagnostics, and patient experiences with hospitals and doctors. Further, campaigns in the media, over the internet, and through the workplace or other institutions, such as general practitioners and hospitals, could be important means by which to inform individuals about their opportunities, rights, institutions, and organizations about which they may otherwise not have known.

Facilitating: The government could arrange the location of facilities for organizations so they are evenly distributed in a community and close to the users or arrange for several organizations to be located at the same place to achieve a mutually supportive environment for the organizations and to create a network among them. For instance, localizing health-related organizations (training groups or support groups) close to a general practitioner's office, a nursing home, or a physiotherapist could increase social capital in the community by reducing transaction costs. Older people could participate in their training more often if the distance to the facility were not farther than walking distance, as then they would not have to rely on others for transportation (Hicks *et al.*, 2011). Participation in voting is widely discussed in the literature.

Health care is also supplied through informal care (van Houtven and Norton, 2004, 2008; Bolin *et al.*, 2008; Bonsang, 2009). To receive and give informal care, such as care for children or help at home, an extensive social network is required for those who are not able to pay for ever service. To adjust for lack of social capital or the ability to pay for services, the government could motivate the construction of voluntary organizations where the aim is to have a large group of people exchanging services between them as well as with individuals who are not able to exchange. Exchanging services implies risk diversification; such organizations are dependent on trust in the community.

Interactions between ISC and CSC

The density of social capital in a community is referred to at the aggregate or community level of social capital. Social capital centers on interaction with others, so one individual's investments in social capital must have an effect on the other individuals in the group network (bonding) or beyond the group (bridging). If the within-group effect of the individual investment in health is more than the sum of the individual investments, then there is a positive externality. A positive externality indicates that even small, individual effects on social capital increase at the aggregate level beyond what is observable for the individual (spillover effects). If the effect of individuals' investments is less than their sum, then there must be some negative effects, such as negative status effects or peer-group effects.

Glaeser *et al.* (2002) predicted the effect of individual investments on the aggregate level, as social capital has a "strong interpersonal complementariness" (Glaeser *et al.*, 2002, p. F443) that could generate positive effects on the aggregate. An implication of this complementarity is a strong social mark-up, a small effect for one individual that may have a large effect on the aggregate, which is often referred to as the social multiplier (Glaeser *et al.*, 2002).

In designing policy, it is important to target policies to investments in social capital that create these positive externalities. Referring to standard economic theory and externalities, the individuals do not incorporate the full benefit of their investments into their investment decisions. Financial incentives equal to the mark-up should be used to adjust for this imperfection.

Bonding and bridging are important concepts in the social capital literature. Bonding refers to increasing effects within a group, while bridging refers to the positive effects of a social network beyond the group itself, such as when a large density of social networks affect an individual even if he/she is not part of the network. A social network could have large positive effects on the group and have a strong bridging effect on some and a negative effect on the others. The bridging effect is a desirable effect that policy makers would like to stimulate, while the bonding effect is undesirable. Not all networks are good for society even when the within-group social capital is very strong; provocative political groups are an example.

Community social capital is sometimes characterized as a "local public good" (Islam *et al.*, 2008). A traditional problem in public economics is free-riding, which occurs when individuals do not reveal their preferences because there are no barriers to accessing and benefitting from the network without investing in it.

Empirical Findings and Policy Implications

There has been extensive research on the effect of social capital on health. The literature contains analyses that measure several health outcomes — general measures like mortality, self-assessed health (SAH), and health-related quality of life (HRQoL), but also channels to health, such as smoking, drinking, other risky behavior, and access to health care. The next links some empirical findings and discusses policies briefly.

Health outcomes

One of the most explicit health outcomes used in the literature is mortality and survival probabilities. (See Islam *et al.*, 2006 for a review.) The finding that social capital affects survival of a particular disease would be very important. Kennelly *et al.* (2003) found no clear indication of this association. More recently, more extended models have been used to show that social capital affects mortality that is due to several causes (Kravdal, 2001; Folland, 2007; Islam *et al.*, 2006; Islam *et al.*, 2008). Hyyppa *et al.* (2007) associated an index for social capital on trust with the mortality of women with cardiovascular diseases. The pathways from social capital should be studied in order to determine what creates the differences. Which types of networks — family, colleagues, friends, or none of these — are the most effective? On the community level, facilitating a high level of social capital could imply positive effects for others in the community. Islam *et al.* (2008) showed that community social capital, such as election rates, affects health-related quality of life, but could not explain the differences between Swedish municipalities.

Several papers have reported the association between social capital (both individual and community) and self-reported health (Iversen, 2008; Rocco *et al.*, 2011; Islam *et al.*, 2006; Poortinga, 2006; see a thorough overview o the main findings in Chapter 3 of this book). The main impression left by the summary of the findings in Chapter 3 is that the association between individual social capital and health is stronger than the one between community social capital and health. As a result, policies should be targeted to give individuals incentives to invest in social capital, such as was discussed in subsection 'Individual Social Capital' (p. 208). However, the review in Chapter 7 provides evidence that individuals with a high return on their investments benefit from a high degree of social capital in the community, that is, there is evidence of bonding. In this situation it is important that policy ensure that groups that fall outside the networks have incentive to invest in social capital. When mental health is studied in detail, such as in Scheffler *et al.* (2007) and Phongsavan *et al.* (2006), the association between social capital and psychological distress is adherent among parents whose children are becoming sick. In that case, it is important for policy makers to ensure the availability of mechanisms that enable parents to maintain their stock of social capital as well as possible. This goal could be accomplished by, for instance, providing paid leave from work or as a publicly funded salary designed for parents with severely ill children.

Channels

Many types of behavior are related to health but are not health outcomes themselves. These behaviors could be defined as channels to health, such as unhealthful behavior (smoking, taking drugs, drinking, and having poor nutrition) and access to healthcare.

Smoking is one of the channels with an unambiguous effect on health, so it is important that policy reduces both the density of smokers and total consumption of cigarettes by smokers. Smoking has been a health outcome in several analyses, and several authors have found a negative association between social capital and smoking (Folland, 2007; Brown *et al.*, 2006, 2011). Married people and individuals in religious groups smoke less than single people and those who are not members of religious groups. A peer-group effect has also been shown to be a factor in smoking behavior (Brown *et al.*, 2006). The peer-group effect makes establishing effective policies trickier, as policies must be targeted to specific individuals in order to change behavior.

Social capital, such as that derived from having a partner or a family, reduces the risk of participation in risky activities because the utility depends on the family's and partner's utility as well. Peer-group effects could have a negative effect on risky behavior as well (Averett *et al.*, 2010; Ali *et al.*, 2011). Averett *et al.* (2010) found that overweight young girls had an increased likelihood of taking part in risky sexual behaviors, so policies must take into account all types of risky behavior.

Traditionally, risky sexual behavior has been related to alcohol consumption, but Markowitz *et al.* (2005) showed that there is no causal relationship between alcohol consumption and the probability of having sex. Therefore, increasing taxes on alcohol will not reduce risky sexual behavior.

Access to high-quality health care is an important factor in producing health, so barriers could create differences in health. As social capital can be an important factor because of the increased information it can provide about possible screening, diagnostic, and treatment options, it is important to determine whether social capital is associated with access to health. In a systematic review of access to health care, the results with regard to the effect of social capital on health were unambiguous (Derose *et al.*, 2009): Among individuals invited to screenings for colorectal cancer, those who lived with a partner or were married were more likely to participate (Aas, 2009). In another analysis, Laporte *et al.* (2008) found a strong relationship between both individual and community social capital and visits to a general practitioner. Networks, measured by peer effects, increase the probability of having a first contact with the health care system (Deri, 2005). Kim *et al.* (2006) analyzed the effect of social capital on physical activity among obese and found no strong association. If more frequent use of health care services reflects the need for health care, policy makers should take measures to reduce the differences. There could be a need to create social networks where information is shared, such as information about the importance of screening. Some studies have shown that women who participate in breast screening have more knowledge about screening guidelines than do women who have had never participated in screening (Bankhead *et al.*, 2003). In the United States, African American women who followed an educational program about breast cancer rates were more likely to attend breast cancer screenings than those who did not follow such a program (Husaini *et al.*, 2001). Hence, education can be an important measure in adjusting for the lack of shared information in families and other networks.

Indexes and policy design

We know that different types of social capital, such as number of friends, number of memberships in organizations, and family situation, correlate and are substitutes. The correlation may vary from setting to setting or for different groups, such as for different types of health outcomes or groups of individuals (e.g., young versus old or men versus women). Therefore, a policy could be effective in one setting but not in another (Eibner *et al.*, 2006). To apply effective policies, a clear understanding of what types of social capital affect health is required in order to target policy. The use of indexes has its advantages empirically, but it could also make the design of policy more complicated, as the true mechanisms may be hidden in the index.

New Types of Networks

Social structures and networks change over time. Travelling, especially by plane, is easier because of lower costs in terms of both prices and time, which could delay or reduce the deprivation of social capital. The increased use of electronic media, such as e-mail, chat, Skype, Facebook, Twitter, and other social or professional networks, also implies changes in social structures. The investment costs for taking part in these networks are low, so it might be easier to stay in contact with friends and connect with other social networks. Electronic media could also work with policy making, as groups and individuals can be reached easily. However, it is important to determine the effectiveness of these networks in promoting health.

Putnam (2000) discussed how the increased use of communication through the internet affects the accumulation and deprivation of social capital. Putnam argued that such communication could be a complement to face-to-face communication, rather than replacing it, writing, "Communication is a fundamental prerequisite for social and emotional connections" (p. 171). However, even though electronic communication cannot fully replace face-to-face communication, one could imagine that, for some groups that face a high cost of entering these networks and are largely isolated from social interactions, the access to networks on the internet reduces barriers that were once present. Facebook has been shown to be associated with increases in bridging social capital (Burke *et al.*, 2011; Ellison *et al.*, 2007). In addition, Burke *et al.* (2011) found that individuals with lower social fluency benefit from these types of connections, even though they are just passively consuming news. Ellison *et al.* (2007) explored the link to health and found an interaction between Facebook use and psychological well-being, especially for users with low self-esteem and low life satisfaction.

Summary and Concluding Remarks

Even though the role of the government in investments in social capital is less important than it is in other investment decisions, financial incentives, regulations, campaigns, and the facilitation of organizations have the potential to be effective measures. However, little is known about the accumulation and deprivation of social capital, which is an important factor in designing policy. Therefore, future research should evaluate the effect of policies on the investment in social capital and on health outcomes.

References

Aas, E. 2009. Pecuniary compensation increases participation in screening for colorectal cancer. *Health Economics*, 18: 337–354.

Aghion, P., Algan, Y., Caluc, P. and Shleifer, A. 2008. Regulation and distrust. National Bureau of Economic Research Working Paper No. 14648.

Ali, M. M., and Dwyer, D. S. 2011. Estimating peer effects in sexual behavior among adolescents. *Journal of Adolescence*, 134(1): 183–190.

Averett, S., Corman, H. and Reichman, N. E. 2010. Effects of overweight on risky sexual behavior of adolescent girls. National Bureau of Economic Research, Working Paper No. 16172.

Bankhead, C. R., Brett, J., Bukach, C., Webster, P., Stewart-Brown, S., Munafo, M. and Austoker, J. 2003. The impact of screening on future health-promoting behaviours and health beliefs: A systematic review. *Health Technology Assessment*, 7(42): 1–92.

Bolin, K., Lindgren, B. and Lundborg, P. 2008. Informal and formal care among single-living elderly in Europe. *Health Economics*, 17(3): 393–409.

Bonsang, E. 2009. Does informal care from children to their elderly parents substitute for formal care in Europe? *Journal of Health Economics*, 28(1): 143–154.

Brown, T. T., Scheffler, R. M., Seo, S. and Reed, M. 2006. The empirical relationship between community social capital and the demand for cigarettes. *Health Economics*, 15(11): 1159–1172.

Burke, M., Kraut, R. and Marlow, C. 2011. Social capital on Facebook: Differentiating uses and users. ACM CHI 2011: Conference on Human Factors in Computing Systems.

d'Hombres B., Rocco, L., Suhrcke, M. and McKee, M. 2010. Does social capital determine health? Evidence from eight transition countries. *Health Economics*, 19(1): 56–74.

Deri, C. 2005. Social networks and health care utilization. *Journal of Health Economics*, 24(6): 1076.

Derose, K. P. and Varda, D. M. 2009. Social capital and health care access. A systematic review. *Medical Care Research and Review*, 68(5): 632–642.

Durlauf, S. 2002. On the empirics of social capital. *The Economic Journal*, 112(November): 459–479.

Eibner, C., and Sturm, R. 2006. US-based indices of area level deprivation: Results from HealthCare for Communities. *Social Science and Medicine*, 62: 348–359.

Ellison, N. B., Steinfield, C. and Lampe, C. 2007. The benefits of Facebook "friends": Social capital and college students' use of online social network sites. *Journal of Computer-Mediated Communication*, 12(4): 1143–1168

Fevang, E., Kverndokk, S. and Røed, K. 2012. Labor supply in the terminal stages of lone parents' lives. *Journal of Population Economics*, 25(4): 1399–1422.

Folland, S. 2007. Does "community social capital" contribute to population health? *Social Science and Medicine*, 64: 2342–2354.

Giordano, G. N. and Lindström, M. 2011. The impact of social capital on changes in smoking behavior: A longitudinal cohort study. *European Journal of Public Health*, 21(3): 347–354.

Glaeser, E. L., Laibson, D. and Sacerdote, B. 2002. An economic approach to social capital. *The Economic Journal*, 112: F437–F458.

Glaeser, E. L., Sacerdote, B. I., and Sacerdote, B. 2002. The social multiplier. *National Bureau of Economic Research Working Paper Series*, Working Paper. 9153, Avaiable at: www.nber.org/papers/w9153.

Grossman, M. 1972. On the concept of health capital and the demand for health. *Journal of Political Economy*, 80(2): 223–255.

Guiso, L., Sapienza, P. and Zingales, L. 2004. The role of social capital in financial development. *The American Economic Review*, 94(3): 526–556.

Guiso, L., Sapienza, P. and Zingales, L. 2008. Trusting the stock market. *Journal of Finance*, 63(6): 2557–2600.

Guiso, L., Sapienza, P., Zingales, L. 2010. Civic capital as the missing link. *National Bureau of Research*, Working Paper No. 15845. Available at http://www.nber.org/papers/w15845.

Hicks, G. E., Benvenuti, F., Fiaschi, V., Lombardi, B., Segenni, L., Stuart, M., Pretzer-Aboff, I., Gianfranco, G. and Macchi, C. 2011. Adherence to a community-based exercise program is a strong predictor of improved back pain status in older adults: An observational study. *The Clinical Journal of Pain*, 28(3): 195–203.

Husaini, B. A., Sherkat, D. E., Bragg, R., Levine, R., Emerson, J. S., Mentes, C. M. and Cain, V. A. 2001. Predictors of breast cancer screening in a panel study of African American women. *Women and Health*, 34(3): 35–51.

Islam, K. M., Merlo, J., Kawachi, I., Lindström, M. and Gerdtham, U. G. 2006. Social capital and health: Does egalitarianism matter? A literature review. *International Journal of Equity in Health*, 5(3), doi: 10.1186/1475-9276-5-3.

Islam, K. M., Gerdtham, U. K., Gullberg, B., Lindström, M. and Merlo, J. 2008. Social capital externalities and mortality in Sweden. *Economics and Human Biology*, 6: 19–42.

Iversen, T. 2008. An explanatory analysis of associations between social capital and self-assessed health in Norway. *Health Economics and Law*, 3: 349–364.

Kennelly, B., O'Shea, E. and Garvey, E. 2003. Social capital, life expectancy and mortality: A cross sectional analysis. *Social Science and Medicine*, 56: 2367–2377.

Kim, D., Subramanian, S. V., Gortmaker, S. L. and Kawachi, I. 2006. US state- and country-level social capital in relation to obesity and physical inactivity: A multilevel, multivariable analysis. *Social Science and Medicine*, 63(4): 1045–1059.

Kravdal, Ø. 2001. The impact of marital status on cancer survival. *Social Science and Medicine*, 52: 357–368.

Laporte, A., Nauenberg, E. and Shen, L. 2008. Aging, social capital, and health care utilization in Canada. *Health Economics, Policy and Law*, 3: 393–411.

Markowitz, S., Kaestner, R. and Grossman, M. 2005. An investigation of the effect of alcohol consumption and alcohol policies on youth risky sexual behaviors. *American Economic Review*, 95(2): 263–266.

Norwegian Ministry of Finance. 2012. For budsjettåret 2013. Skatter, avgifter og toll 2013 (For the 2013 Budget. Taxes, fees and customs 2013. Prop. 1LS2012–2013).

Phongsavan, P., Chey, T., Bauman, A., Brooks, R. and Silove, D. 2006. Social capital, socio-economic status and psychological distress among Australian adults. *Social Science and Medicine*, 63(10): 2546–2561.

Poortinga, W. 2006. Social capital: An individual or collective resource for health? *Social Science of Medicine*, 62: 292–302.

Putnam, R. D. 1993. The prosperous community: Social capital and economic growth. *American Prospect*, 4(13): 35–42.

Putnam, R. D. 2000. *Bowling Alone: The Collapse and Revial of American Community*, New York: Simon & Schuster.

Rocco, L., Fumagalli, E. and Suhrcke, M. 2013. From social capital to health and back. *Health Economics* (forthcoming).

Scheffler, R. M. and Brown, T. T. 2008. Social capital, economics, and health: New evidence. *Health Economics, Policy and Law*, 3: 321–331.

Scheffler, R. M., Brown, T. T. and Rice, J. K. 2007. The role of social capital in reducing non-specific psychological distress: The importance of controlling for omitted variable bias. *Social Science & Medicine*, 65: 842–854.

Scheffler, R. M., Brown, T.T., Syme, L., Kawachi, I., Tolstykh, I., and Iribarren, C. 2008. Community-level social capital and recurrence of acute coronary syndrome. *Social Science & Medicine*, 66: 1603–1613.

Tabellini, G. 2008. The scope of cooperation: Values and incentives. *Quarterly Journal of Economics*, 3: 905–950.

van Houtven, C. H. and Norton, E. C. 2004. Informal care and health care use of older adults. *Journal of Health Economics*, 23(6): 1159–1180.

van Houtven, C. H. and Norton, E. C. 2008. Informal care and Medicare expenditures: Testing for heterogeneous treatment effects. *Journal of Health Economics*, 27(1): 134–156.

Index

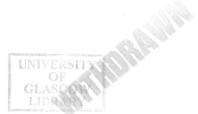